MANAGING
TRAUMATIC STRESS RISK

MANAGING TRAUMATIC STRESS RISK

A Proactive Approach

By

DOUGLAS PATON, PH.D., C. PSYCHOL.

*School of Psychology, University of Tasmania
Launceston, Tasmania, Australia*

JOHN M. VIOLANTI, PH.D.

*Department of Criminal Justice
Rochester Institute of Technology, Rochester, New York
School of Public Health and Health Professions
State University of New York at Buffalo, New York*

CHRISTINE DUNNING, PH.D.

*Department of Governmental Affairs
University of Wisconsin, Milwaukee, Wisconsin*

and

LEIGH M. SMITH

*School of Psychology, Curtin University
Perth, Western Australia*

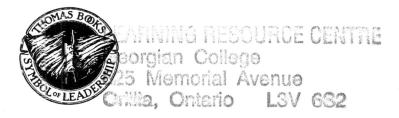

CHARLES C THOMAS • PUBLISHER, LTD.
Springfield • Illinois • U.S.A.

Published and Distributed Throughout the World by

CHARLES C THOMAS • PUBLISHER, LTD.
2600 South First Street
Springfield, Illinois 62704

©2004 by CHARLES C THOMAS • PUBLISHER, LTD.

ISBN 0-398-07517-4 (hard)
ISBN 0-398-07518-2 (paper)

Library of Congress Catalog Card Number: 2004046027

With THOMAS BOOKS *careful attention is given to all details of manufacturing
and design. It is the Publisher's desire to present books that are satisfactory as to their
physical qualities and artistic possibilities and appropriate for their particular use.*
THOMAS BOOKS *will be true to those laws of quality that assure a good name
and good will.*

Printed in the United States of America
UB-R-3

Library of Congress Cataloging-in-Publication Data

Managing traumatic stress risk: a proactive approach / by Douglas Paton . . . [et al.].
   p. cm.
Includes bibliographical references and index.
ISBN 0-398-07517-4 – ISBN 0-398-07518-2 (pbk.)
   1. Job stress. 2. Post-traumatic stress disorder–Prevention. 3. Stress management. 4.
Employee health promotion. 5. Hazardous occupations–Psychological aspects. 6. Emergency
management–Psychological aspects. 7. Disasters–Psychological aspects. 8. Work–
Psychological aspects. I. Paton, Douglas.

HF5548.85.M364 2004
158.7'2–dc22
                                                                                2004046027

CONTRIBUTORS

Paul T. Bartone, Ph.D., received his Ph.D. in Psychology/Human Development from the University of Chicago in 1984. Since 1985, he has served as a research psychologist for the U.S. Army, first at the Walter Reed Army Institute of Research (WRAIR) in Washington, D.C., then as Director of the WRAIR psychology field unit in Heidelberg, Germany, and more recently as a research scientist, Department of Behavioral Sciences and Leadership, United States Military Academy, West Point. He is presently assigned to Industrial College of the Armed Forces at the National Defense University, Washington, DC. He has conducted numerous studies of stress, health and adaptation among military personnel and their families. He serves as member-at-large for the Military Psychology Division (19) of the American Psychological Association and also chairs that division's Committee on International Military Psychology.

Jacquie Bicknell lectures in the Masters of Health Counselling at Curtin University of Technology, Perth, Western Australia. Her interest in traumatology originated in her earlier forensic work and is reflected in her psychology honors research on Secondary Traumatic Stress in therapists working with the perpetrators of sexual abuse. Jacquie's interests now extend to the relevance of posttraumatic growth for trauma therapists, which is a focus of her Ph.D research investigating the negative and positive transformations experienced by therapists in their trauma work. Prior to entering academia, Jacquie was with the Western Australian Department of Justice for eight years. Her forensic work included assessment, therapeutic program delivery, and program review for the male perpetrators of sexual abuse.

Christine Dunning, Ph.D., is a professor and Chair of the Department of Governmental Affairs at the University of Wisconsin–Milwaukee. She received her Ph.D. in Criminal Justice/Social Science from Michigan State University. In addition, she attended Marquette University Law School. Dr. Dunning formerly served as Associate Director–Police at the Des Moines, Iowa, Criminal Justice Center and as Director of In-Service Police Training for Southeastern Wisconsin Police Academy. She has published extensively on police stress and trauma, on disaster stress management, and in numerous areas of police administration. She consults with officials responsible for mitigation in a large number of catastrophic events annually.

Anne Gehrke is a candidate for a graduate degree in Psychology Studies at the University of Technology, Dresden, Germany. Her specialization is in occupational health psychology, and her major interests are in police, trauma, and posttraumatic stress disorder (PTSD). Anne recently completed an internship with the Rochester, NY, Police Department PD, which provided her with good insight into the everyday experiences of police officers in the field. She was assigned to the police academy, to various patrol sections, to Technicians, Child Abuse, Homicide, Forgery, and Frauds Units. Anne also took part in "significant others" meetings and police mental health training; worked with victim assistance; participated in Juvenile Accountability Conferencing (JAC), in S.A.F.E. Kids (a program for traumatized children), and in a Community Volunteer Response Team, which detects persons at risk of PTSD after a homicide occurs in their residential area. Anne has taken courses in CISM, trauma, and PTSD, as well emergency psychology. Her goal is to complete the additional education in emergency psychology as a special qualification, working with police and maybe other occupational groups who are confronted with emergency situations, and to focus on secondary prevention of trauma and PTSD as an aspect of occupational safety and health.

Kathryn Gow, Ph.D., is a Senior Lecturer in the School of Psychology and Counselling at the Queensland University of Technology. She has been the inaugural Coordinator of the Clinical Hypnosis program and the new Graduate Diploma in Mental Health, and teaches about trauma in the postgraduate courses, and manages a large postgraduate supervision cohort. She has worked voluntarily with Australian Vietnam Veterans in many aid programs in Vietnam receiving awards from the Vietnamese government and the QUT for her community service activities. She has worked as a psychologist in private practice and acted as a consultant to several large corporate training programs. Her conference papers and publications range across many fields with stress, burnout, and trauma being an area of ongoing interest.

Greg Hannan, Ph.D., is currently Senior Lecturer in Psychology at the University of Tasmania. He has been interested in applied organizational settings since 1989, when he became involved in selection and training of air traffic controllers in Australia. He completed his Ph.D. in the area of air traffic controller selection and validation in 1999 and has worked on several major projects involving the evaluation of human factors issues in complex workplace settings, including Airservices Australia, Tasmania Police, Comalco Bell Bay, and TEMCO. Among his interests in these fields are person-environment fit and the relationship between cognitive workload and situation awareness in complex socio-technical systems.

Colleen McFarlane is training to be a clinical psychologist and is enrolled in a Ph.D. program at Monash University, Melbourne, Australia. Her Ph.D. dissertation is an investigation of stress, trauma, and resilience among international and national humanitarian aid workers. Her research interests include the relationship of traumatic stress to war and civil conflict, the role of psychology in "developing" nations, psychology across cultures, refugee studies, and the development of qualitative research methods within psychology. Her clinical experience has been with refugees and asylum seekers, children with developmental delay and mental illness in Cambodia, young people suffering from psychoses, women suffering from eating disorders, and people who have experienced life-threatening medical conditions.

Douglas Paton, Ph.D., is an Associate Professor in the School of Psychology at the University of Tasmania, Australia. He is the founding editor of the *Australasian Journal of Disaster and Trauma Studies*. He has written extensively on stress and traumatic stress in emergency services and emergency management groups and consults on staff and organizational development of emergency organizations. His current research is concerned with the longitudinal analysis of stress in police services, stress in incident commanders and other disaster response personnel, and stress in urban search and rescue groups.

Stephanie Samuels has served and is presently serving as a consultant for police agencies in matters of psychological concern. In addition, she has her own private practice. She has conducted debriefing of officers involved in emotionally charged incidents who are experiencing symptoms of PTSD. She has worked with legislators in changing the workman's compensation laws to cover psychological injuries. She is responsible for the initiation of a Law Enforcement Officers Hotline in the State of New Jersey. Her responsibilities included designing policies and procedures, community outreach, hiring of staff, and recruiting and evaluating volunteers and support staff. She has been involved in designing volunteer training manuals, implementing training, assessing equipment, and overseeing the budget of the hotline. Stephanie has designed and implemented workshops on suicide prevention, emotional survival after a critical incident, PTSD, domestic violence, emotionally disturbed people, and alcohol and divorce prevention for all recruits going through the police academy. She has conducted in-service police training on emotionally disturbed people, sexual harassment, racial bias, and stress management.

Eugene Schmuckler, Ph.D., is Coordinator of Behavioral Sciences/Management at the Georgia Public Safety Training Center. He received his B.S. degree from Brooklyn College in psychology and his M.A. and Ph.D. degrees from Louisiana State University in industrial/organizational psychology. Dr. Schmuckler is a member of the International Society for Traumatic Stress Studies and the Association of Traumatic Stress Specialists (ATSS). He has served on the board of directors of ATSS and was editor of the association's newsletter, *Trauma Lines.* Dr. Schmuckler is a diplomate in police psychology and is a certified trauma specialist.

Peter Sevastos, Ph.D., is coordinator of the Masters program in Organizational Psychology at Curtin University of Technology, where he also teaches units in occupational stress and human resources management. His current research interests are in the areas of job-related affective well-being and job satisfaction, organizational commitment and organizational citizenship behavior, and the examination of gender issues at work.

Jane Shakespeare-Finch, Ph.D., is a lecturer in the School of Psychology at the University of Tasmania in Australia. Her primary research focus is in understanding and promoting positive posttrauma changes, particularly in the context of emergency service work. Jane has published book chapters and articles in this area of study. She teaches in a number of areas including psychological research methods, health psychology, trauma, personality and positive psychology. Her research focuses on positive changes that result from the experience of a traumatic event and on the role of personality and coping factors in predicting posttrauma outcomes Current research addresses vicarious trauma in emergency service work and the catalyst such events can provide for posttraumatic growth.

Leigh M. Smith M.A., is Head of the School of Psychology at Curtin University of Technology in Perth, Western Australia. His main research foci are the development and application of research techniques and data analysis in applied settings, measurement theory, and the construction of psychological response scales. He is interested in psychological well-being at work and, in particular, the relation between organizational practices and the mental health of workers.

A. J. W. Taylor is an Emeritus Professor of Psychology at Victoria University of Wellington with a continuing interest in stress/trauma research stemming from his adolescent days in the bombing of London to a concern for the welfare of the emergency personnel involved in the recovery of body parts after the 1979 aircrash of Mt. Erebus and more recently to Pacific Island communities after a cyclone, a tragic school dormitory fire, and to a political coup and hostage-taking. He has attempted to formalize his observations and clinical experience in numerous papers, and he extends his findings here to the occupational stress that civilian and military peacekeepers face.

John M. Violanti, Ph.D., is a Full Professor at the Rochester Institute of Technology (RIT), Rochester, New York, and an Associate Research Professor at the University of Buffalo School of Public Health and Health Professions, Department of Social and Preventative Medicine. Dr Violanti has focused the majority of his work on police trauma, suicide, and health concerns. He is the author and coauthor of numerous journal articles and eight other books on those topics.

PREFACE

Traumatic stress has long been thought of as an occupational hazard in protective services professions. This thinking has resulted in such occupations frequently being described as "high-risk" professions. Although such professions may indeed be at risk for traumatic events in their work, this exposure does not necessarily mean that individuals will experience negative outcomes as a result. In this text we argue that the presumption of "risk" as defining negative pathological outcomes due to trauma exposure is misleading. We offer a less prescriptive definition of risk, one that affords protective services organizations a framework within which they can proactively develop strategies to increase the positive and reduce the negative consequences of trauma and disaster work. Indeed, the inevitable, regular, and repetitive nature of traumatic exposure in the professions covered in this book calls for this approach if organizations are to effectively discharge their duty of care.

DOUGLAS PATON
JOHN M. VIOLANTI
CHRISTINE DUNNING
LEIGH M. SMITH

CONTENTS

MANAGING
TRAUMATIC STRESS RISK

Chapter 1

TRAUMATIC STRESS: PERSPECTIVES ON MANAGING RISK

Douglas Paton, John M. Violanti, Christine Dunning,
and Leigh M. Smith

INTRODUCTION

Traumatic stress has long been recognized as an occupational hazard in protective service professions. Recognition of their status in this regard has resulted in their frequently being described as "high risk" professions. In this text we argue that this use of risk is misleading, particularly in regard to its presumption of an automatic association with negative and pathological outcomes. Here a less prescriptive definition of risk is offered, one that affords protective service organizations a framework within which they can proactively develop strategies to increase the positive and reduce the negative consequences of trauma and disaster work. Indeed, the inevitable, regular, and repetitive nature of traumatic exposure in the professions covered in this book calls for this approach if organizations are to effectively discharge their duty of care.

RISK MANAGEMENT

Although typically associated with loss, risk also encompasses the concepts of choice, anticipation, and resilience (Hood & Jones, 1996). According to this conceptualization, the risk concept is a future-oriented one capable of accommodating perspectives that cover adaptational, growth, and distress outcomes. Importantly, it implies an ability to make choices in regard to how personnel (through, for example, selection, training, and support) will interact with threatening events to influence the likelihood of their experiencing positive or negative outcomes. It thus represents a comprehensive basis for traumatic stress management in professions regularly and repetitively exposed to challenging and dangerous work.

Risk is a product of the interaction between the frequency of occurrence of adverse events and the consequences of such exposure. It is difficult to influence the frequency of exposure; protective services professionals must respond to events that are unpredictable in regard to, for example, their timing, nature, duration, and location. However, we can make choices in regard to the consequences of this exposure. In the risk equation, consequences are represented by an interaction between hazards (e.g., stressors, operational and environmental demands) and the resilience resources mobilized to deal with them.

In regard to its application to traumatic stress management, risk management is concerned with estimating levels of loss or growth outcomes likely following exposure to a specific event. It does so by anticipating the consequences likely to ensue when the characteristics of personnel (linked to selection, training, experience) and organizational systems and procedures interact with the characteristics of specific critical incidents. From such analyses, risk management policies can be developed and appropriate practices and strategies implemented. Collectively, this will encompass a range of related activities for identifying and assessing risk, developing and implementing risk reduction interventions, and monitoring and evaluating their effectiveness. It is an iterative process that improves planning by contributing greater insight into the implications and consequences of different decisions and courses of action. Risk management affords opportunities for priority setting based on providing the greatest degree of risk reduction using the available resources.

The foundation upon which the attainment of these objectives is based is risk analysis. Risk analysis encompasses risk assessment and risk evaluation. A key element here is risk assessment, comprising hazard assessment and resilience and vulnerability assessment. Risk assessment provides the raw material for evaluating the likely consequences of exposure to particular events. This approach is fundamental to the pursuit of the goal of promoting resilient personnel. Specifically, it is necessary to identify the hazards to understand what people and systems must be resilient to.

Resilience resources were discussed in a previous volume (Paton, Violanti, & Smith, 2003). Here we are concerned with articulating the event and organizational factors that arise when responding to incidents, the psychological hazards. This provides the foundation for the systematic examination of how specific outcomes (e.g., growth, adaptation, loss) arise and, consequently, what resilience resources are required to facilitate positive outcomes. From this analysis, appropriate risk management policies, procedures, and practices can be developed.

In applying a risk management approach to traumatic/disaster stress management, the hazard component of the equation will be represented by the environmental and situational characteristics and demands capable of threatening psychological equilibrium. It is on the identification, analysis and assessment of hazards and the contexts in which they arise that this volume will concentrate.

HAZARD ANALYSIS AND RISK REDUCTION

Psychological hazard analysis is complicated by the fact that hazards are difficult to discern from a consideration of the event per se. The hazard is not the air crash, the hostage situation, or the terrorist bombing. Rather, hazards are the event characteristics and operational demands that can threaten psychological equilibrium. For example, hazards could be exposure to large-scale death and serious injury, handling human remains, being prevented by the scale or complexity of an event from employing one's professional expertise, having to make urgent and complex decisions, inadequate response resources, and so on. Furthermore, the implications of these characteristics will be influenced by contextual factors (e.g., interaction with specific organizational practices, the work-family interface). Consequently, systematic and comprehensive risk management must go beyond the analysis of the demands likely to be encountered in a specific emergency and anticipate how contextual factors (e.g., from family and operational practices and systems) influence traumatic stress risk. Importantly, a focus on articulating these characteristics within the risk assessment process increases the likelihood of personnel being able to adapt to a range of events.

It is important to note that we are not denying the fact that the hazards encountered when responding to a critical incident or disaster can threaten the psychological equilibrium of those who respond to it. We do argue that the threat to psychological equilibrium, if analyzed within the conceptualization of risk adopted here, is not prescriptive in regard to the personal (or organizational) consequences of this exposure. Rather, it identifies the starting point for estimating the consequences for personnel and the actions that can be taken to facilitate positive outcomes and minimize negative outcomes. In other words, we can make choices in regard to whether the challenge to psychological equilibrium is resolved through adaptation or growth, or through diminished capacity and distress.

By providing a systematic review of the hazards capable of eliciting traumatic and disaster stress in emergency professionals, this volume provides information on one part of the risk management equation. Integrating this knowledge with that on resilience resources provides a framework for developing more comprehensive models of the traumatic stress process in protective service professions and for proactive planning organizational risk management policy and practices capable of facilitating well-being and growth and minimizing distress.

This volume provides a systematic review of critical incident and disaster hazards, the contextual factors that influence risk, and their implications for traumatic stress risk management. This knowledge is fundamental to planning how to facilitate adaptive and positive resolution in personnel facing the prospect of repetitive exposure to hazardous or adverse operational demands. Risk management provides a mechanism with which organizations can estimate the capability of their personnel to deal with hazardous and adverse work experiences, and develop this capability to facilitate both the execution of their duty of care and their role in protecting the community. Here we argue that this goal can be accomplished through the systematic integration of strategies involving, for example, selection, training, support, and organizational change and development. The systematic assessment of this capability and continued attention to its development will substantially increase the capacity of protective service professionals to deal with the emergencies and disasters that are all too frequent facets of their working lives.

CHAPTER CONTENT

This volume presents a systematic review of hazards associated with trauma and disaster work intended to facilitate the proactive management of traumatic stress risk. Collectively, the contributions provide a broad overview of hazards (e.g., handling human remains or making decisions in high pressure situations) and the contextual factors that influence their consequences (e.g., family demands, operational demands such shift work, bureaucracy, and socio-legal demands from the criminal justice system).

The first three chapters explore several issues fundamental to understanding risk across a range of protective service populations. Following a brief discussion of the nature of traumatic stress, Schmuckler, in Chapter 2, outlines a temporal framework for conceptualizing and planning risk management strategies. In particular, he introduces the need to expand thinking beyond the response phase, which is the focus of most studies, to consider how mobilization and recovery present their own unique risk factors.

An historical focus on postevent intervention has limited the attention paid to the choices available in regard to the predispositions of those employed in emergency and law enforcement professions. In Chapter 3, Dunning discusses selection from a sociolegal perspective, particularly in regard to identifying the competencies that can direct the process of developing selection practices that reconcile legal compliance with the selection of people capable of operating in complex and threatening environments. She then proceeds to review the existing psychometric tests that could be employed in this context. The theme of identifying appropriate procedures is continued in Chapter 4 where Smith provides an innovative overview of issues that must be tackled when assessing protective behaviors capable of influencing risk.

The text then switches to a discussion of risk factors within specific professions. This section commences in Chapter 5 with Samuels' discussion of how developmental history can represent a risk factor for police officers. In Chapter 6, Gehrke and Violanti continue the discussion of risk in police officers, but explore it from an operational perspective. Protective service professionals face a range of hazards that change as they progress through the stages of disaster response. The implications of these stages for traumatic stress risk are reviewed by Paton and Hannan in Chapter 7.

Increasing involvement of the international community in the management of the consequences of war and civil unrest has resulted in the traditional role of the military personnel being supplemented by a need for them to perform in a peacekeeping capacity. The risk factors associated with the reconciliation of these roles are discussed by Bartone in Chapter 8. Then, in Chapter 9, Paton, Taylor, and McFarlane discuss stress risk in humanitarian aid contexts.

The risk status of the above professional groups can be traced to their direct exposure to dangerous and adverse circumstances. For some professions, risk arises from the need for them to exercise their professional responsibilities in regard to meeting the needs of those directly affected by trauma and disaster. In Chapter 10, Bicknell discusses risk of secondary or vicarious trauma in therapists and counselors.

In addition to its being attributed to demands associated with a critical incident or disaster, risk is also influenced by several contextual factors. In the final section, three such influences are discussed. Like all employees, protective service professionals work within organizations characterized by, for example, culture, regulations, procedures, and management practices. Growing evidence for the influence of such characteristics on both positive and negative outcomes following exposure to specific critical incidents requires that organizational factors be included within traumatic stress risk management planning. Sevastos, in Chapter 11, reviews this issue. The discussion of contextual factors is continued in Chapter 12, where Shakespeare-Finch and Gow discuss how the work-family interface influences traumatic stress risk. The events of September 11, 2001, resulted in the spectre of terrorism being firmly embedded in the landscape of traumatic stress. The issue of terrorism is discussed by Violanti in Chapter 13. Although the hazards encountered when responding to the consequences of a terrorist attack are similar to those discussed in preceding chapters, the nature of terrorism means that response takes place within a very unique context, justifying the specific consideration of its influence within the risk management process.

REFERENCES

Hood, C., & Jones, D. K. C. (1996). *Accident and Design: Contemporary Debates in Risk Management.* London: UCL Press.

Paton, D., Violanti, J. M., & Smith, L. M. (2003). *Promoting Capabilities to Manage Posttraumatic Stress: Perspectives on Resilience.* Springfield, IL: Charles C Thomas.

Chapter 2

MENTAL HEALTH CONSIDERATIONS
FOLLOWING A DISASTER

EUGENE SCHMUCKLER

"But I don't want to go among mad people," Alice remarked.
"Oh, you can't help that," said the cat:
"We're all mad here. I'm mad. You're mad."
"How do you know I'm mad?" said Alice.
"You must be," said the cat, "or you wouldn't have come here."
Lewis Carroll, *Alice in Wonderland*

THE NATURE OF DISASTER

Disaster and trauma are not new phenomena. Flooding and metropolitan destruction were recorded in the book of Genesis (chapters 6 and 7). Pepys described his own nightmares subsequent to the 1666 Fire of London (Daly, 1983). The attack and destruction of the World Trade Center (WTC) in 2001, because of its real-time television coverage, significantly increased the attention focused on disasters and their sequelae. The dramatic magnitude of this disaster extended its impact well beyond the population immediately affected. This tragedy, however, represents only one disaster in a string of like events. Between 1967 and 1991, disasters around the world killed 7 million people and affected 3 billion (Cater, Revel, Sapir, & Walker, 1993).

To a greater or lesser extent, natural, technological, and human-made disasters share common elements – speed of onset, suddenness, unexpectedness – resulting in a swath of physical and human destruction. The speed of onset of a disaster limits opportunities for those in its path

9

to emotionally prepare for the impact. While each disaster holds the potential of impacting those immediately affected (e.g., bystanders, rescue workers, the immediate community), some disasters, such those at Lockerbie, Chernobyl, Piper Alpha, Bhopal, Bosnia, and the World Trade Center, create an impact that ripples across national and international borders.

There is no one definition of a disaster. Korver (1987) identified over 40 definitions in the literature. In general, the term denotes an event causing widespread damage and suffering sufficient to warrant supplementing state and local efforts to mitigate damage, loss, hardship or suffering (Federal Emergency Management Agency [FEMA], [1994]).

There are also a number of schemas for classifying disaster depending upon cause, effect, number of injuries and deaths, degree of personal impact, nature of illnesses generated in the aftermath along with other epidemiological data (Figley, Giel, Borgo, & Harotis-Fatouros, 1995). Regardless of schema used, the following criteria apply:

1. A disaster disrupts the existing social structure making it difficult for the usual social mechanisms to manage the consequences. It needs to be understood that difficulties resulting from disasters are many and are not limited solely to those that are of a physical nature.

2. Variables that moderate the impact of disasters include the ability of survivors to adjust psychologically, the capacity of the human structures to adapt to the crisis, and the amount of support available.

3. Groups that have been subjected to the prolonged need to cope with disasters, as might be experienced in developing countries, may become part of a disaster "subculture" affecting patterns of psychosocial reactions to the disaster situation (Raphael & Newman, 2000).

The overall impact of a disaster is a function of its cause, particularly whether it was of natural or human origin. Natural disasters such as hurricanes, tornados, and earthquakes are generally seen as being unavoidable. Nevertheless, they have the potential of causing significant physical destruction, social disruption, and loss of home and income (Weisaeth, 1995). Disasters of human origin, such as toxic chemical and nuclear accidents, dam collapse, transport accidents, explosions, hostage taking, mass gathering incidents, war and terrorism, particularly when involving acts of commission or deliberate malfeasance, are particularly likely to result in survivors' experiencing or perceiving a loss of control, which leads them to seek a scapegoat. (Raphael & Newman, 2000).

Recent occurrences of chemical, radiological, and biological terrorism; the release of Sarin gas in Japan; the Chernobyl meltdown; and the anthrax attacks in the United States add a new dimension to disasters attributed to human action. The physical or physiological responses resulting from attacks of this nature may approach epidemic proportions (Di Giovanni, 1999). The loss of control experienced as a consequence reiterates the role of the origin of a disaster as a significant stress risk factor.

WHO IS AFFECTED?

Disasters affect individuals across a broad spectrum without regard to age, gender, ethnicity, or national origin albeit at differential levels. In addition, disasters affect persons on the basis their proximity, physically and emotionally, to the disaster event. Taylor and Frazer (1982) describe six categories of victims:
- Primary victims: Those directly exposed to the catastrophic event.
- Secondary victims: Grieving relatives and friends of the primary victims.
- Third-level victims: Those who respond professionally.
- Fourth-level victims: The community involved in the disaster, including those who converge, who altruistically offer help, who share the grief and loss, or who are in some way responsible.
- Fifth-level victims: People who, even though not directly involved with the disaster, may still experience states of distress or disturbance.
- Sixth-level victims: Those who, but for chance, would have been primary victims themselves, who persuaded others to the course that made them victims, or who are in some way indirectly or vicariously involved.

Although Taylor and Frazer present the categories in a linear fashion, they conceptualize impact as a series of asymmetric circles linked by the ripple effect. In regard to level three, groups likely to be affected include search and rescue workers (including dogs); fire and safety workers; transport drivers; medical personnel and paramedics; medical examiner and staff; police, security, and investigators; clergy; and mental health and social service personnel, along with volunteers. Although all may be involved in the same disaster, differences in personality, professional affiliation, and patterns of involvement can create a unique risk context for each group. Risk must also be assessed relative to the phase of involvement.

RISK AND DISASTER EXPOSURE

Just as there is no one definition or type of disaster, it is unrealistic to think of risk in a prescriptive manner. While some risk factors, such as the magnitude of loss (deaths, numbers of injured), severity of impact, recurring danger, and threat to life (Figley et al., 1995), appear to be pervasive, risk is more aptly conceptualized in a contingent manner. In regard to these contingent influences, meaning and the phase of involvement are prominent factors.

EMERGENCY WORKERS AND THEIR RESPONSES

Individual responses to disasters are a direct function of the meaning that the individual attaches to the event. Regardless of cause, natural or man-made, the disaster events are different (having their own unique characteristics), disruptive, and dangerous. The differences stem from the fact that the event is something with which the individual is not prepared by either experience or training to cope. How many persons have made the comment, "Just when you think you have seen it all along comes something totally different"? As this chapter was being written, on February 1, 2003, newscasts detailed the loss of the Columbia shuttle with its entire international crew of astronauts. Imagine the difficulty in a training environment to simulate the smell of a single burn fatality, let alone the massive number that might be encountered in a major explosion.

The disruptive aspect is that the event itself alters the normal day-to-day routine of the individual. It has a sudden onset, and the disruptions are unpredictable. The event gains control of the person's life usually for an extended period of time. The result is that the individual becomes a victim of the disruptive event. There is also a perceived (as well as real) danger to the individual, to someone the individual loves or cares for, or to some valued possession or activity. The person believes that there is a real risk of loss involved as the result of experiencing the crisis event.

DISASTER PHASES

Raphael and Newman (2000) identify five phases of disasters: preparation and planning; threat and warning; impact; immediate post-disaster; and recovery phase. Each phase, while not necessarily clearly delineated, has its own implications for the assessment of risk and its consequences.

In the preparation and planning phase, whose relationship with the onset of action is indicated by color-coded warnings ranging from a low-threat condition (green) to one that is severe (red), individuals (civilian, military, and emergency workers) receive education about possible disaster experiences. This training will include likely psychological reactions and ways in which to deal with them. This form of predisaster inoculation provides disaster workers with tools to recognize and deal with postdisaster stress effects.

In addition to direct effects, stress risk during the impact phase is affected by the "illusion of centrality." This term describes the person who feels as if he or she is the only one being affected. Off-duty fire fighters, police officers, emergency medical technicians (EMTs), and medical personnel respond to disaster situations even though they may have the day off or have just completed a shift. Rescue workers report feelings of dissociation as they perform their duties. Some persons feel paralyzed or stunned and may experience the "freeze" component of the general stress response.

During the 18 to 36 months following the event, the recovery period, a predictable pattern of behaviors is exhibited. These behaviors have been referred to as the heroic honeymoon, disillusionment, and re-stabilization phases. The heroic phase is characterized by individuals and the community directing inordinate levels of energy into the activities of rescuing, helping, sheltering, emergency repairing, and cleaning up. The increased physiological arousal and behavioral activity can last from a few hours to a few days. For emergency personnel these efforts result in their working extended lengths of time and not wanting to be pulled off the assignment.

The second phase, the honeymoon phase, which lasts up to three months, is one of optimism and camaraderie. This fellowship is evidenced by individuals, strangers before the event, befriending, housing, and feeding others affected by a common event. Dignitaries appear on the scene offering support and encouragement along with promises of assistance. Entire groups of persons, especially disaster workers, become media celebrities.

Within a relatively short time the attention of the media and the world is focussed on other areas and situations. The disaster scene becomes yesterday's news. Fatigue, irritating experiences, and the knowledge of all that is required to restore lives to some form of normalcy produce disillusionment. The complexity of rebuilding becomes all too apparent. At that point, individuals question why others are receiving more recognition than them. Long-simmering grievances begin to be voiced in the form of complaints regarding betrayal, abandonment, lack of justice, bureaucratic read tape, and general incompetence. Disaster workers may begin complaining that one group is receiving a disproportionate amount of praise and glory.

The fourth stage, reconstruction, begins when individuals regain equilibrium. It occurs within 6 months for some and up to 36 months for others, if it does in fact occur. It is during this time that rescue workers often decide that they are ready to find other types of employment.

EFFECTS OF TRAUMATIC STRESS IN
A DISASTER SITUATION

Paton (1994) discusses impact in terms of the involvement of professionals whose disaster role may bear superficial similarity to their routine role. Paton justifies the latter by drawing a distinction between technical expertise and psychological preparedness, with the latter being challenged by the extreme and atypical nature of the demands encountered.

Hartsough (1985) observes three major sources of stress for disaster workers: emergency occupations, the events and hazards confronting workers in disasters, and the organizational and social context of the work they do. Kling (1988) has pointed out that civilian and worker survivors of a disaster are affected somewhat differently. During the impact stage it is not unusual for individuals to experience "peritraumatic" stress symptoms. Symptoms occur during or immediately after the traumatic disaster experience. Among these symptoms are dissociation, intrusive reexperiencing, avoidance, hyperarousal, anxiety, depression, problematic substance abuse, and psychotic symptoms. The people at greatest risk for extreme peritraumatic stress include those who experience life-threatening danger; extreme loss or destruction of their homes, normal lives, and community; intense emotional demands for distraught survivors; as well as those with prior psychiatric or marital/family problems and prior significant loss, such as death of a loved one in the past year.

The length to recovery depends on predisaster functioning, the characteristics of the event (situational variables), the victim's professional role, and organizational variables (Hartsough, 1985). Following a review of the literature, Norris, Friedman, Watson, Byrne, Diaz, and Kaniasty (2002) conclude that an adult's risk for psychological distress increases as the number of the following factors increases:

- Female gender
- 40 to 60 years old
- Little previous experience or training relevant to coping with disaster
- Low socioeconomic status
- Children present in the home
- For women, the presence of a spouse, especially if he is significantly distressed
- Psychiatric history
- Severe exposure to the disaster, especially injury, life threat, and extreme loss
- Living in a highly disrupted or traumatized community
- Secondary stress and resource loss.

Event characteristics involve elements such as number of survivors, terrain and weather, the media, and the number and ages of bodies. Exposure to the psychological trauma of an incident increases the likelihood of post-situation stress. When rescuers have a personal relationship with the victims, they will register higher stress levels. Responding to the Gander military air disaster, participants frequently reported personal identification with the dead soldiers and the tendency to think, "It could have been me." In addition to the stress of exposure to burned and mutilated bodies, personal identification was a contributing risk factor for increased stress (Bartone, 1985).

Disaster workers capable of identifying strongly with their professional role during a rescue task suffer fewer long-term stress symptoms. When the professional role of the disaster worker cannot be maintained adequately, the risk of adverse outcomes increases. In the case of the Gander air disaster, the horror, difficulty, and sheer exhaustion experienced by workers in the mortuary resulted in emotional and behavioral changes in many participants. Bartone (1985) notes that these symptoms and reactions occurred in both professionals and inexperienced volunteers, and questions whether it would be possible for any amount of training or experience to adequately prepare workers to deal with large numbers of dead bodies.

Organizational actions, particularly in regard to decisions or operational procedures, may contribute to the disaster worker's stress risk. The agency can be a source of protection, comfort, and support against the hazardous effects of disaster work, but inappropriate practices and decisions contribute to negative outcomes.

Stress responses are in fact a normal reaction (Frankl, 1959). Mild-to-moderate stress reactions during the emergency and early postimpact phases of disaster are prevalent because rescue workers accurately recognize the grave danger in disaster (Young, Ford, Ruzek, Friedman, & Gusman, 1988). Although stress reactions may seem "extreme" and cause distress, they generally do not become chronic problems. It would be unusual for an individual who has been affected by a disaster not to show some form of emotional distress. Mild-to-moderate stress reactions are seen during the impact and early postimpact phases of the disaster with the majority of persons fully recovering within six to sixteen months (Baum & Fleming, 1993; Green & Lindy, 1994; Steinglass & Gerrity, 1990). Following a disaster, most child and adult survivors experience one or more of the following normal stress reactions for several days:

- Emotional reactions – temporary feelings of shock, fear, grief, anger resentment, guilt, shame, helplessness, hopelessness, or emotional numbness. The latter reaction is shown by survivors who experience difficulty feeling love and intimacy or difficulty taking interest and pleasure in day-to-day activities.
- Cognitive reactions – confusion, disorientation, indecisiveness, worry, shortened attention span, difficulty concentrating, memory loss, unwanted memories, and self-blame.
- Physical reactions – tension, fatigue, edginess, difficulty sleeping, bodily aches or pain, startling easily, racing heartbeat, nausea, change in appetite, and change in sex drive.
- Interpersonal reactions in relationships at school or work, in friendships, in marriage, or as a parent; distrust; irritability; conflict; withdrawal; isolation; feeling rejected or abandoned; being distant judgmental, or over-controlling.

Most disaster survivors only experience mild, normal stress reactions. However, as many as one out of every three disaster survivors experience some or all of the following severe symptoms which may lead to posttraumatic stress disorder (PTSD), anxiety disorders, or depression:

- Dissociation (feeling completely unreal or outside yourself, as in a dream; having "blank" periods of time you cannot remember). Many disaster workers actually use this technique as a coping mechanism when confronted with overwhelming situations.
- Intrusive reexperiencing (terrifying memories, nightmares, or flashbacks).
- Extreme attempts to avoid disturbing memories (through self-medication or substance abuse).
- Extreme emotional numbing (completely unable to feel emotion, as if empty).
- Hyperarousal (panic attacks, rage, extreme irritability, intense agitation).
- Severe anxiety (paralyzing worry, extreme helplessness, compulsions, or obsessions).
- Severe depression (complete loss of hope, self-worth, motivation, or purpose in life.

For some individuals, risk is increased by their interpretation of their experiences that manifests itself in the form of guilt. Opp and Samson (1987) describe five types of guilt: survivor, demonic, moral/spiritual, betraying/abandoning, and superman. Demonic and moral/spiritual guilt are most likely to be found among military personnel who have been involved in combat situations.

> They are the blessed. They are also the burdened. They are the 17 men and women who walked safely down from the upper reaches of the south tower of the World Trade Center on Sept. 11. For each of them, every new day is a gift, but one that carries an implicit question: Why me? (Eric Lipton, *New York Times*, June 2)

"It is fresh in my mind," said one survivor from the 84th floor. "I went to war, and I didn't ask to go. I wasn't prepared for it. I wasn't trained for it." And then he posed the question, "Why did I live?"

It is understandable that civilians, the nontrained, might experience this feeling. Yet many disaster workers share the same set of emotions, those associated with survivor guilt. Those experiencing survivor guilt hold the feeling that it is they who should have died, that they do not deserve to live, and that somehow their survival has cheated someone out of living. As a result, many survivors believe they have an obligation to live for that other person; if they get to the point where they view their own life as a failure, they believe they have failed the other person. The principal effect is a sense of unworthiness, and the behavior pattern reflects a fear of success. These individuals tend to sabotage events just when things are going well. They can be indifferent to living, sometimes with poor personal maintenance and hygiene. They often experience periods of extreme risk-taking behavior, pushing their safety to the limits, which is not a desirable behavior pattern for disaster workers.

Betraying/abandoning guilt stems from the survivors' sense of not having done enough for those they have been sent to recover or help. Being unable to respond to a coworker's cry for help or to uncover a buried survivor quickly enough may be viewed as a shameful failure. Individuals with this type of guilt experience shame. They feel a strong sense of regret, moral anguish, and personal responsibility for having committed a breach of conduct. Such individuals will look small, stay slumped in their seat, and maintain poor eye contact. Because of their perceived failure, leaving the profession is not unlikely.

Superman guilt stems from disaster workers' believing they have superhuman capabilities, are able to see in the dark, or have some other type of sixth sense. They believe these extraordinary qualities could have enabled them to prevent the situation that occurred. As a result of the disaster having taken place, they carry a profound sense of failing others as well as themselves at a vital time. Media coverage focusing on errors in response to the situation can exacerbate this guilt. Individuals with this guilt feel personally responsible but helpless in the face of their human limitations. The principal effect is a sense of failure. Rescue workers with this type of guilt become overly controlling in their personal relationships in an effort to control all of the variables so that their significant others or children or employees will be safe. Another behavioral response is for them to actively abdicate all responsibility and avoid intimate relationships or employment where they might be placed in positions in which they again would have responsibility for others.

It is important to recognize that many individuals demonstrate a number of positive responses in the aftermath of disaster. These include altruism (helping save or comfort others), relief and elation at surviving disaster, the sense of excitement and greater self-worth, changes in perception of the future, and interpretations of experiences in ways that contribute to psychological growth (Paton, Violanti, & Smith, 2003).

POST DISASTER

No one who experiences a disaster is untouched by its impact. Although exposure produces emotional shock and may cause many emotional problems, they are a normal response to an abnormal situation. No two individuals will be affected in a similar way.

It is difficult to understand disasters without considering the need to give meaning and inner form to the experience and to life thereafter (Lindy, 1993). Hodgkinson and Stewart (1991) suggest that the survivor's search to understand the experience of the disaster exists on a number of levels, a "hierarchy of formulation." They propose the following chronological sequence.

1. When did it happen?
2. How did I escape?
3. Why did I escape?
4. Why do I feel like this?
5. What does the way I feel now mean about me as a person?
6. What does all that I have been through mean about the way I understand life?

Through recognition of the impact of disaster, it is possible for the affected individual to minimize its long-term consequences. To relieve the stress and strain imposed by the attack on the World Trade Center and its aftermath, the New York Police Department (NYPD) ordered all 55,000 of its employees, including uniformed employees, to attend mental health counseling. This decision by the NYPD to mandate counseling follows the program implemented for rescue workers after the Oklahoma City bombing in 1995 (Orner, 2000). Ironworkers who were involved in the rescue and salvage operations subsequent to the events of September 11, 2001, have turned to a federal screening program run by Mount Sinai School of Medicine to get help with both physical and mental problems. As one worker stated, "It's over, but it's not over. You were working in a graveyard and saw a lot of stuff you weren't meant to see, and a lot of it still lingers. We talked to each other all the way through the cleanup, and we're still doing it."

Complicating personal recovery is the prevalence of a mind set defining the disaster worker as being a tough survivor. Brende (1993) describes "The 12 Commandments of Tough Survivors":

1. Though shalt be powerful as steel, not flesh.
2. Though shalt not be confused by outsiders.
3. Thou shalt stand alone.
4. Thou shalt reveal nothing which stains your image.
5. Thou shalt show only tough meanness.
6. Thou shalt not reveal fear.
7. Thou shalt not admit fault.
8. Thou shalt not cry.
9. Thou shalt not acknowledge vulnerability to death or death wishes.
10. Thou shalt get even.
11. Thou shalt never relax, acknowledge defeat, or give up.
12. Thou shalt not request affection, warmth or love.

Dr. Robin Herbert, codirector of the World Trade Center Worker and Volunteer Medical Screening Program, says that many workers from 9/11 suffer from respiratory problems and psychological difficulties, including posttraumatic stress disorder. She calls the workers "the invisible walking wounded."

Despite these after-effects, the tendency is for disaster workers not to seek out help. Although disaster workers have a high capacity for trust among themselves, they tend to be uncertain about the competencies of outsiders. Disaster workers may demonstrate mental and emotional resilience during an operation but have intense emotional reactions afterwards because of their sensitivity to the feelings of survivors and their families. These qualities make it difficult for them to seek help from others who are not seen as being part of the rescue worker family.

There are also substantial data to suggest that disaster workers will not seek out services, despite reporting significant emotional distress (Sprang, 1999). Indicative of the need for postdisaster interventions is data showing that although not restricted to disaster workers, nearly half of those individuals directly exposed to the Oklahoma City bombings had an active postdisaster disorder, with PTSD being diagnosed in approximately one-third (North et al., 1999).

The personal recovery of the individual is a direct function of the coping mechanisms used by the rescue worker. Coping mechanisms may be categorized as being cognitive, emotional, and coping. These coping strategies are described in Table 2-1.

TABLE 2-1
CATEGORIES OF COPING MECHANISMS

	Positive Coping	**Negative Coping**
Cognitive	• Logically analyzing impact • Trying to prioritize efforts and needs • Mentally rehearsing • Options – Making decisions using coping and imagery	• Avoiding thoughts • Forgetting it happened • Denying the impact • Having wishful thoughts • Experiencing self-attribution or self-blame
Emotional	• Accepting and tolerating • Experiencing a range of emotions • Regulating emotions through cognitive or physical means	• Suppressing emotions • Having emotional outbursts • Misdirecting feelings • Feeling resignation/fated • Waiting for time to help
Problem-focused coping	• Seeking assistance • Developing plans • Looking at life style and balance	• Engaging in drinking, drugs acting out • Sinking into passivity • Engaging in overacting

Developed by Dr. Betsy Gard.

Organizational factors can play a critical role in postdisaster recovery and thus should be accommodated within risk management strategies. Subsequent to a disaster, the following organizational factors can influence traumatic stress risk:

1. Routine workload requires continued attention while role conflict and discomfort increase as a result of new and competing demands.

2. Routine management procedures are ruptured, and tolerance among departments and personnel often decreases as stress, role conflict, and extreme fatigue set in.

3. Limited credit may be given if emergencies are handled effectively; harsh judgments may increase if emergencies are handled poorly.

4. Increased media scrutiny of procedures may increase risk for traumatic stress.

5. Increased scapegoating as personnel seek to relieve anxiety may occur.

6. Disruption and increased stress results in a decrease in managers' ability to see the "big picture."

Various techniques for dealing with postdisaster situations have been developed, including that of critical incident stress debriefing (CISD) (Mitchell, 1993). A common theme of CISD debriefing is its role in normalizing feelings. It is far from being the sole approach. Raphael (1993) emphatically takes the position that CISD is not appropriate for everyone and should never be mandatory. Orner (2000) has found that there is no "uniformity of need" and that the majority of participants need to be given the option of receiving CISD rather than having it imposed on them by organizational structure. A need for more systematic evaluation has also been stated (Rose & Bisson, 1998). Along with the response to the immediate disaster event, individuals bring to a disaster a history of predisaster stress and organizational stressors.

Other approaches to managing postdisaster stress risk include cognitive behavioral therapy (CBT), exposure therapy, cognitive therapy, and stress-inoculation training. Exposure therapy entails disaster workers' describing their traumatic experiences in detail, repetitively, to reduce the arousal and distress associated with their memories. Cognitive therapy focuses on helping survivors to identify their trauma related negative beliefs (e.g., guilt and distrust of others) and to change them in order to reduce distress. Stress-inoculation training teaches patients skills for managing and reducing anxiety using techniques such as breathing, self-relaxation, and positive self-talk.

Organizations seeking to mitigate traumatic stress risk should consider the implementation of appropriate training (pre- and post-disaster). They should also consider team work (preferably using a buddy system, with the less experienced teaming up with one who is more experienced); ready availability of on-scene support (physical and psychological); limitations of shifts and breaks as required; and clear roles and responsibilities in line with personal and professional capabilities.

Disaster workers experience reactions similar to those of the general population, such as stress reactions, feelings of helplessness, high arousal, guilt depression, and posttraumatic stress disorder. Along with these negative reactions, disaster workers also may experience a sense of achievement and positive self-worth.

Follow-up and specialized counseling may be required for disaster workers who experience persistent problems. If this counseling is in fact the desired course of action, organizational backing is critical so that the affected worker does not feel inadequate.

Regardless of structure, culture, and needs, rescue organizations should establish outreach services (such as those offered by employee assistance programs [EAPs]); expect and prepare to address an increase in problems related to substance abuse, marital and family dysfunction, and financial concerns; offer screening for primary, secondary, or tertiary victims; and encourage managers (this may require training) to know the impact of the disaster on their staff in order to provide specific support. Some key indicators of this impact include employees with injured relatives; employees who have had to relocate; an increase in work-related accidents; an increase in tension among employees or departments; significant changes in job productivity; and more discussion of leaving the profession.

With the passage of time, recovery issues for rescue workers include working out an understanding of the event; reestablishing a new equilibrium/life; reestablishing trust; and reestablishing a future. During the recovery process, families and friends become cosurvivors. The disaster worker may find that anniversaries of the event bring all the memories back and induce posttrauma feelings. Posttrauma feelings will decrease in intensity and frequency with appropriate treatment, but will not completely go away. And finally, survivors must recognize that their lives will be changed forever.

REFERENCES

Bartone, P. (1985). *The Human Response to The Gander Military Air Disaster: A Summary Report.* Washington, DC: Department of Military Psychiatry, Division of Neuropsychiatry, Walter Reed Army Institute of Research.

Baum, A., & Fleming I. (1993). Implications of psychological research on stress and technological accidents. *American Psychologist, 48,* 665–67.

Brende, J. O. (1993). A 12 step recovery program for victims of traumatic events. In J. P Wilson & B. Raphael (Eds). *International Handbook of Traumatic Stress Syndromes* (pp. 867–877). New York: Plenum Press.

Cater, N., Revel, J., Sapir, D., & Walker, P. (1993). *World Disasters Report 1993.* Geneva: The International Federation of Red Cross (IFRC) and Red Crescent Societies (RCS).

Daly, R. J. (1983). Samuel Pepys and post-traumatic stress disorder. *British Journal of Psychiatry, 160,* 309–314.

Di Giovanni, C. (1999). Domestic terrorism with chemical or biological agents: Psychiatric aspects. *American Journal of Psychiatry, 156,* 1500–1505.

Federal Emergency Management Agency. (1994). *Community Emergency Response Team: Participant Handbook.* A publication of FEMA. Emergency Management Institute and the National Fire Academy. *FEMA Workbook for Developing an Application for Crisis Counseling Services for Disaster Victims.*

Figley, C., Giel, R., Borgo, S., Briggs, S., & Harotis-Fatouros, M. (1995). Prevention and treatment of community stress: How to be a mental health expert at the time of disaster. In S. E. Hobfoll & M. W. de Vries (Eds.), *Extreme Stress and Communities: Impact and Intervention* (pp. 489-497). London: Kluwer Academic Publishers.

Frankl, V. E. (1959). *Man's Search for Meaning.* New York: Touchstone Press.

Gard, B. (2003). Personal Correspondence, Atlanta, GA.

Green, B. L., & Lindy, J. D. (1994). Post-traumatic stress disorder in victims of disasters. *Psychiatric Clinics of North America, 17,* 301–309.

Hartsough, D. M. (1985). Disaster Work and Mental Health: Prevention and Control of Stress Among Workers. Rockville, MD: Center for Mental Health Studies of Emergencies, U.S. Department of Health and Human Services.

Hodgkinson, P. E., & Stewart, M. (1991). *Coping with Catastrophes. A Handbook of Disaster Management.* London: Routledge.

Kling, E. A. (1988). Factors related to the appraisal of stress in firefighters. *Dissertation Abstracts International, 49* (B), p. 4008.

Korver, A. J. H. (1987). What is a disaster? *Prehospital and Disaster Medicine, 2,* 152–153.

Lindy, J. D. (1993). Focal psychoanalytic psychotherapy of post-traumatic stress disorder. In J. P. Wilson & B. Raphael (Eds.), *International Handbook of Traumatic Stress Syndromes* (pp. 803–810). New York: Plenum Press.

Lipton, E. (2001, April 19). In Cold numbers: A census of September 11 victims. *The New York Times,* p. 3.

McFarlane, A. C. (1995). Stress and disaster. In S. E. Hobfoll & M. W. de Vries (Eds.), *Extreme Stress and Communities: Impact and Intervention* (pp. 287–314). London: Kluwer Academic Publishers.

Mitchell, J. T. (1993). Traumatic stress in disaster workers and emergency personnel: Prevention and intervention. In J. P. Wilson & B. Raphael (EDs), *International Handbook of Traumatic Stress Syndromes* (pp 905–914). New York: Plenum Press.

Norris, F., Friedman, M. J., Watson, P.J., Byrne, C. M., Diaz, E., & Kaniasty, K. (2002). 60,000 disaster victims speak: Part 1: An empirical review of the empirical literature. *Psychiatry: Interpersonal and Biological Processes, 65*(3), 207–239.

North, C. C., Nixon, S. J., Sariat, S., Mallonee, S., McMillen, J. C., Spitznagel, E. L., & Smith, E. M. (1999). Psychiatric disorders among survivors of the Oklahoma City bombing. *JAMA, 282,* 755–762.

Opp, L. E., & Samson, A. Y. (1987). *A Taxonomy of Guilt for Combat Veterans.* Presented at the 3rd Annual Meeting of the Society for Traumatic Stress Studies, New Orleans, LA.

Orner, R. J. (2000). *Points of Controversy in the Debriefing Debate and the Search for a New Evidence Base for Early Intervention after Trauma.* Paper presentation at the Third World Conference for the International Society for Traumatic Stress Studies. Melbourne: ISTSS

Paton, D. (1994). Disaster relief work: An assessment of training effectiveness. *Journal of Traumatic Stress, 7,* 275–288.

Paton, D., Violanti, J. M., & Smith, L. M. (2003). *Promoting Capabilities to Manage Posttraumatic Stress: Perspectives on Resilience.* Springfield, IL: Charles C Thomas.

Pynoos, R. S., Steinberg, A.M., & Wraith, R. (1995). A developmental model of childhood traumatic stress. In D. Chicchetti & D. Cohen (Eds.), *Manual of Developmental Psychopathology. Vol. 2: Risk, Disorder and Adaptation* (pp. 72–95). New York: Wiley.

Raphael, B. (1993). *Disasters Management.* Canberra: Australian Government Publishing Service.

Raphael, B., & Newman, L. (2000). *Disaster Mental Health Response Handbook*. New South Wales: Institute of Psychiatry.

Rose, S., & Bisson, J. (1998). Brief early psychological interventions following trauma: A systematic review of the literature. *Journal of Traumatic Stress, 11*(4), 697–710.

Sprang, G. (1999). Post disaster stress following the Oklahoma City Bombing: An examination of three community groups. *Journal of Interpersonal Violence, 14,* 169–183.

Steinglass, P., & Gerrity, E. (1990). Natural disasters and post traumatic stress disorder: Short-term versus long-term recovery in two disaster-affected communities. *Journal of Applied Social Psychology, 20,* 1746–1765.

Taylor, A. J. W., & Frazer, A. G. (1982). The stress of post-disaster body handling and victim identification. *Journal of Human Stress, 8,* 4–12.

Weisaeth, L. (1995). Preventive psychosocial intervention after disaster. In S. E. Hobfoll & M. W. de Vries (Eds.), *Extreme Stress and Communities: Impact and Intervention* (pp. 410–419). London: Kluwer Academic Publishers.

Young, B. H., Ford, J. D., Ruzek, J. I., Friedman, B. J. & Gusman, F. D. (1988). *Disaster Mental Health Services: A Guidebook for Clinicians and Administrators*. St. Louis, MO: National Center for PTSD, Department of Veteran Affairs Employee Education System.

Chapter 3

REDUCING PROTECTIVE SERVICE WORKER TRAUMA THROUGH PREEMPLOYMENT SCREENING

CHRISTINE DUNNING

INTRODUCTION

The field of risk management in workplace safety has almost universally come to accept the potential for mental injuries in employees and "customers" of organizations experiencing workplace crime, violence, accident, and disaster. Assumptions regarding the relationship between traumatic events and mental injury in these contexts have resulted in acceptance for the need for some type of program to forestall such negative consequences. Action has been limited to logistical planning, audits of potential for traumatic events, and the adoption of internally- or externally-delivered protocols for debriefing programs. The expectation that individuals involved in traumatic events need to be seen immediately by a mental health professional has permeated societal belief systems, especially after media coverage of such events as the two World Trade Center terrorist events.

This is especially true in the protective services. Police, fire, corrections, and disaster and emergency medical organizations have embraced the concept of mental injury to their staff due to trauma being as much a risk as physical injury when responding to crime, violence, accident, and disaster. Yet most intervention programs have been based on reactive protocols initiated by some identified threshold event such as a shooting or major fire incident. This critical incident structure belies the fact that what is seen as traumatic is highly individual. It assumes that trauma is the result of a "group" experience and that the intervention should use the same structure to resolve the event. Individual experience interventions, especially when they involve the "small" or "anomalous" trauma not apparent to others but to the individual affected, have no such initiating response. It is expected that the individual employees seek the services of an employee assistance program (EAP) for their personal trauma experiences, much as has always been the case in the history of the profession. But experience clearly tells us that this does not generally happen. Relief is not sought privately, except in ways that ultimately can prove destructive to career and individual. Turning to the bottle, misuse of prescription medications, or physical presentations in the form of illness or injury have been associated with traumatic work experiences in the protective services for decades.

Of course, it is inappropriate to assume that all protective service workers exposed to critical incidents are traumatized or even stressed. One must first recognize and accept that demanding events can equally produce *eustress* − "good stress." Frequently, those who experience trauma report its positive effect on their lives. The assumption that traumatic exposure produces trauma, or even stress, ignores the reality that many individuals value their traumatic event as a learning and growth experience. Nor does any administrator want to intentionally contribute to the stress, trauma, or ineffectiveness of their workers, especially after the harrowing experience of a traumatic event. Concern for trauma mitigation and worker safety remains of utmost importance in the management of trauma workers. Understanding how to react and proceed with both informal and formal responses to trauma management has resulted in the establishment of reactive intervention models for trauma experience as the standard of practice in most trauma mitigation organizations. This chapter presents a new role for clinicians, that of providing proactive assessment of trauma resilience as part of the screening/hiring process. The reader is asked to think outside the traditional structure of the reactive therapeutic treatment experience and to recognize other proactive roles and tasks that must be accomplished to mitigate the psychological impact of trauma experience associated with work-related events. Specifically, the mental health clinician/practitioner is being asked to develop skills to serve as a management consultant to assist administrators to select stress/trauma hardy individuals or, at the minimum, to determine training needs to instill resiliency in their newly selected employees.

There is no doubt that work organizations today are experiencing the impact of sudden destruction and chaos, unprecedented violence, accident, crime, and disaster. Increasingly, they are finding that Employee Assistance and conventional human resources consultants may not be equipped to deal constructively with larger psychological issues that underpin and promote successful readjustment to traumatic events. As administrators increasingly seek the services of consultant psychotherapists and those trained in systems/group counseling to resolve their problems of impact on organizational climate, employee performance, and personnel issues, they have embraced traditional clinical psychologists and psychotherapists as having a role in organizational consultation.

To date, most clinicians have responded by providing their basic skills associated with "talk therapy" to attempt to address the damage and injuries that befall employees, employers, and the entire organization subsequent to a workplace catastrophic or traumatic event. Martin (1996) asserts that the transition can be difficult and complex for most clinicians trained in the rituals and values of private practice. Schooled in diagnosis and assessment for pathology and in techniques of treatment, many psychologists are ineffective because they lack the fundamental knowledge and understanding of the role of psychology in organizations. In contrast, industrial-organizational and consulting psychology do possess the theoretical, practical, and research validation for applying psychological concepts to the workplace, work group, and employee to protect those in high-risk traumatic stress-exposed occupations and to prevent or reduce injury from deployment in traumatic work situations.

PROTECTIVE WORKER SELECTION

In today's employment climate, human capital has become an increasingly expensive commodity that requires management beyond the "original purchase." Personnel selection and retention that involves ensuring a best fit between the person, the job, and the organization have become as costly as the labor costs of performing the duties of the job. Selection is critical when the worksite and work duties involve high risk for personal physical and mental injuries, conditions that are inherent in the work of employees in police, fire, corrections, emergency medical, and disaster mitigation organizations.

The best-equipped protective service agency is only as good as the competence of its personnel. This means that one must select those who can perform the duties of the position and maintain that competency in the face of extreme stress and danger. In addition, the ability of the worker and the organization to recover after experiencing a high-risk, critical incident is also paramount. Administrators must ensure that only highly capable, hardy individuals are permitted to serve such organizations. Failure to do so only results in poor service and potential harm to the community and to the staff as well. Therefore, administrators of protective service agencies must be aware of the factors involved in such competencies, such as stress resilience, and they must select personnel best suited to withstanding both routine and adverse demands of the job, just as they now do by setting physical condition standards to reduce the occurrence of physical injuries.

The selection process for those in the protective services has changed greatly over the last two decades as mandates occasioned by case and statutory law, societal demands for accommodation, and the labor pool have changed. Managers know that the success of their organization depends on the quality of personnel not only to "do the job" but also to "withstand the rigors of the job." Quality of service is not the only indicator of a good selection process. The attrition rate due to duty-incurred disability, disciplinary attrition, and the costs associated with impaired workers also affect work product. As a consequence, a human resource objective of protective service agencies needs to incorporate a process by which candidates can be screened for their "resiliency or stress-resistance" hardiness as a bona fide occupational qualification.

This is not to say that such consideration has not historically occurred in the protective services. To an extent, even though not stated as an explicit goal, administrators have utilized criteria that serve to select stress-hardy employees. For example, the requirement of a minimum age, overtly set to meet legal standards for being able to take an oath or hold a permit to carry a weapon, has been set at 18. Where once new protective service employees were predominantly hired at an age closest to the minimum (to maximize years of service from each candidate), organizations now tend to hire older, more experienced and mature individuals. Educational standards have also been raised. Where minimum standards were once set at the lowest level of completion, generally of secondary education (high school diploma or equivalent), most agencies now require two or more years of higher or more specialized educational attainment. Successful completion of a basic course of study, either through an academy, basic training course, or certification workshop, has become more complicated as these programs have grown in length of time commitment and rigor of curriculum. Successful applicants thus tend to have higher intelligence, greater motivation, and more focused commitment to successful employment. They are also able to present documentation of their ability to undergo and successfully cope with the stress associated with study, mastery, testing, and standard attainment.

Good moral character is determined by a thorough background investigation, which involves the applicant's being fingerprinted (for comparison against local, state, and federal criminal records); having his or her financial/credit history examined, driving and education records reviewed, and employment history checked; and allowing interviews with past friends, colleagues, neighbors, and teachers. This information is used to discern an ability to cope with stress. Biodata (Table 3-1) have been used for decades in the selection process. This character investigation, one of the most expensive and time-consuming steps in the entire selection process, has always been considered the most important element of the selection process. However, it is also considered to be the most subjective and conducive to discrimination against some classes of persons without being able to justify its use against a bona fide occupational standard. So important is the accuracy of this data that some agencies have used the polygraph and/or psychological stress evaluator to determine the veracity of the applicant's report of such information.

TABLE 3-1
SAMPLE BIODATA ITEMS

• Personal data	• Motor vehicle records
• Marital status and former marital status, including divorces, annulments, or widowhood	• Unemployment and disability records
• Educational background	• Financial history
• Military service	• Adult criminal and juvenile record
• International travel	• History of drug and alcohol use
• Selective service status	• Loyalty oath
• Employment record	

The hiring process itself is stressful, and candidates unable to cope with the process indicate their inability to meet the rigor of the stress of the job. Candidates with poor educational, employment, financial, personal behavior, or relationship histories tend to be eliminated. One could assert that elimination of these applicants from the pool of potential hires screens out poor stress copers. Those with existing stress conditions or injuries or with poor coping skills have some kind of negative impact in their personal, occupational, or social functioning. It is assumed that independently of how much stress an individual may have been under in his or her past, poor management of stress leaves behind a trail in an individual's ability to learn, work, relate, behave, or conform. Maintaining a good personal record in the face of life's trials is evidence enough of stress coping skills.

This is especially true for the occupations considered here. The protective services also place great emphasis on past military service. Veterans' preference points virtually assure employment for those with prior military service records. For example, veterans comprised almost 100% of the hires during the 1960s to almost the end of the 1980s. The preference for veterans has changed legally over time. The law provides veterans' preference points for individuals who have been in active service of the United States during a recognized war period or other recognized conflicts as defined by federal law. (At one time, military service itself, with honorable discharge, sufficed for applicants to receive the preference.) Veterans' preference points are added to the final score and may improve a veteran's position on the list of qualified candidates. Any eligible veteran who claims preference has five points for service and 10 points, if claiming a disability, added to his or her final passing examination score. This applies both to written examinations and to training and experience. Veterans' preference does not mandate an interview or guarantee employment, but the added five points always result in these candidates topping the hiring list, especially for civil service positions.

While each state, and country in the case of Canada and Australia, holds different standards for applying veterans' preference points, the reality is that new hires in the 1970s and 1980s were predominantly military combat veterans. Veterans of more recent conflicts in Beirut, Panama-Grenada, Desert Storm, and now Eastern Europe, Afghanistan, and Iraq also benefited from the preference. The protective services were able to select from a pool of potential candidates who had extensive experience in dangerous and life-threatening situations, had documented stressful work conditions, and still had relatively unblemished personal records, evidencing a capacity to deal with stress. Having survived combat mentally and behaviorally unscathed, the candidate could probably survive police work.

Since the late 1980s, the number of applicants for protective service positions who possess such a preference status has markedly declined. Candidates are now more likely to come out of an educational institution than to have served in the armed forces. Moreover, candidates are more likely to be women who have no experience in competitive team contact sports, another frequent source of injury-threat experience. Biodata from these candidates do not provide as many clues about their ability to handle stress, nor do they indicate personal coping strategies, or suggest resiliency or hardiness. As a result, police departments, recognizing that police officers would be placed under moderate-to-severe stress, began to use some form of psychological screening around 1970 (International Association of Chiefs of Police, 1973). The understanding that officers handle arrests when surrounded by hostile crowds, attacks, and assassinations of officers, the recognition of the possibility for mental injuries through exposure to critical incidents like shootings, accidents, and violence, as well as the acknowledgment of the relationship of such exposures to acts of police violence, misuse of alcohol and prescription drugs, self-medication with illicit drugs, and emotional instability, provided departments with the legitimacy to use psychological screening in legal occupations.

Psychological instruments have been used to a varying extent throughout the United States for police applicant screening since 1917 (Territo, Swanson, & Chamelin, 1977). Although long criticized for problems related to properties of validity, reliability, standardization, and utility, a few standard tests now are extensively used in police and fire selection. The selection process of interest here is the use of personality testing and its ability to predict stress-resistance, management, coping strategy, and resiliency. Personality is a series of constructs or inferences that can be derived from observations of behavior of selection of preferred responses. The field of personality profiling has been rigorously researched internationally because component traits of personality are not only difficult to define but also difficult to measure. People differ on many psychological and physical characteristics. These characteristics are called *constructs*. Constructs cannot be seen or heard, but we can observe their effects on other variables. Professionally developed tests and procedures that are used as part of a planned assessment program are designed to select more qualified and productive employees. However, it is essential to understand that *all assessment tools are subject to errors,* both in measuring a characteristic (e.g., verbal ability) and in predicting performance criteria (e.g., success on the job). The appropriate use of professionally developed assessment tools on average enables organizations to make more effective employment decisions than the use of simple observations or random decision-making.

Personality inventories have a long history of use in police, fire, and correctional agencies. They are less costly, are less time-consuming, and have fewer problems with reliability and validity than do the generally accepted personality inventories now in use. Starting with the use of the Minnesota Multiphasic Personality Inventory (MMPI) in the late 1960s, departments now accept their findings as providing guidance in selecting from among a pool of candidates. In 1978, the Equal Employment Opportunities Commission (EEOC) and three other federal agencies – the Civil Service Commission (predecessor of the Office of Personnel Management) and the Labor and Justice Departments – jointly issued the *Uniform Guidelines on Employee Selection Procedures.* The *Guidelines* incorporate a set of principles governing the use of employee selection procedures according to applicable laws. They provide a framework for employers and other organizations for determining the proper use of tests and other selection procedures.

The *Guidelines* are legally binding under several civil rights laws, including Executive Order 11246, the Civil Rights Requirements of the National Job Training Partnership Act, and the Wagner Peyser Act. In reviewing organizational testing practices under Title VII, the courts generally give great importance to the *Guidelines'* technical standards for establishing the job-relatedness of tests. They apply to all tests, inventories, and procedures used to make employment decisions. The *Guidelines* do not require that employers show the job-relatedness of the assessment procedures. However, it strongly encourages the use of only job-related assessment tools, especially since Title I of the Civil Rights Act (CRA) of 1991 specifically requires demonstration of both the job-relatedness and business necessity of assessment instruments or procedures that cause adverse impact under the Americans with Disabilities Act (ADA) – 1990. A qualified individual with a disability is one who can perform the essential functions of a job, with or without reasonable accommodation.

The Americans with Disabilities Act (ADA) – 1991 precludes the use of psychological tests that diagnose pathology in preemployment screening. Therefore, agencies cannot use tests that diagnose the existence of posttraumatic stress disorder (PTSD) on candidates before a job offer is proffered and accepted. Nor can they use any other test that screens for any mental health pathology in preemployment. Psychological tests must relate to a specific job-related competency. Law enforcement agencies are under an especially heavy obligation to improve their techniques for detecting the high-risk candidate before hire. A high-risk candidate is one whose total psychological make-up is such that the candidate will likely be unable to cope with the responsibilities and authority inherent in the position of police officer. Early in the use of psychological tests, the focal area of competency was emotional stability, generally involving the use of the Eysenck Personality Inventory comprised of a battery of perceptual tests that looked at three major personality traits: emotional stability versus neuroticism; extroversion versus introversion; and realism versus psychoticism.

The utility of personality inventories in employee selection for protective services workers who might suffer a traumatic stress injury lies both in determining a work-related competency that can meet the test of being a bona fide occupational qualification and the fact that they represent a psychological test which can validly measure that construct without diagnosing pathology. Examinations used in police organizations for personnel selection include the MMPI-2 (Minnesota Multiphasic Inventory-2 PSY 5), the CPI (California Personality Inventory), the TJTA (Taylor-Johnson Temperament), and IPI (Inwald).

JOB COMPETENCIES AND RISK FOR POSTTRAUMATIC STRESS DISORDER

The first question the consultant must address is whether there is a competency related to traumatic stress, stress resiliency, and emotional stability that can be accepted as being job-related to the protective services whose work exposes officers to high risk for the development of traumatic stress. The issue is to develop labels of competency to capture what would be required of a good worker with abilities to withstand and respond to such conditions, then to find a test that measures those constructs.

The management of stress involves such variables as developmental factors of the personality, exposure experience, and learned ability or dysfunction as the result of experiencing stress. These variables suggest that the competency profile must include information about personality as it relates to stress, data on lifetime stress and trauma exposure, and information about coping style and strategies.

The task of the consultant is to operationalize the competency related to resiliency to stress. Competencies are those characteristics of an individual which underlie performance or behavior evidenced at work. (Slivinski, Loremore, & Miles, 1997). By developing a list of competency concepts or labels, the consultant can link performance to success on the job. Since personality for the individual tends to be consistent across time and situations, a personality test that mirrors the competency related to stress and resilience can provide the employer with information about the candidate's potential to perform in a high–trauma-exposure environment. Five general dimensions of personality have been identified repeatedly in the literature (Barrick & Mount, 1991; Costa & McCrae, 1992; Digman, 1990; Goldberg, 1994; McCrae & John, 1992). The Five Factor Model (FFM) or "Big Five" approach has emerged as the dominant taxonomic approach in personality research (Digman, 1990). Although FFM critics exist (Block, 1995), many researchers and practitioners have adopted the common framework provided by the FFM (Costa & McCrae, 1995; Goldberg, 1993; McCrae & John, 1992). In applied use, FFM constructs have been shown to be valid predictors of a wide variety of criteria (Paunonen & Ashton, 2001). In particular, industrial-organizational psychologists have produced a large body of research examining the predictive relationships between FFM personality dimensions and job performance (Barrick & Mount, 1991; Hurtz & Donovan, 2000; Mount & Barrick, 1995; Salgado, 1997).

In this model, personality is evident in five contexts: social, interpersonal, goal or work-related, emotional, and experiential. Of interest is the emotional orientation – those behaviors evident in emotional contexts such as stress and frustration. In regard to emotional orientation, tendencies and preferences for behaviors include tolerance for stress/frustration and resilience. The predictability and range of emotional response are also aspects of emotional orientation. Traditionally, stress has been described in more physical competencies such as the psychosocial capacities of resistance to stress, energy, health, vigilance, selective attention, and stamina.

The consultant must determine which of the various personality tests with sufficient validity and reliability in construction and predictability and that include competency constructs for stress, resiliency, and tolerance can be used in personnel selection to screen candidates for the protective services. In addition, consultants must review other screening criteria that might be used to flag potential for resilience or decline in candidates when they are placed in traumatic work situations. In order to accomplish these tasks, the consultant must first consider which preconditions have been empirically linked to increased risk for traumatization.

RISK FACTORS FOR POSTTRAUMATIC STRESS DISORDER

Although the *Diagnostic and Statistical Manual of Mental Disorders* (American Psychiatric Association, DSM-IV-TR, 2000) conceptualizes posttraumatic stress disorder as a learned response to a severe event that involves a subjective affective component, empirical research suggests that the probability of occurrence is also related to the severity, duration, and proximity of exposure (direct learning factors). It also can involve predisposing risk factors (Shalev, 1996; Yehuda, 1999a) that may or may not be learned and the type of traumatic event experienced (Davidson & Foa, 1991; Kessler, Sonnega, Bromet, Hughes, Nelson, & Breslau, 1999; McFarlane & de Girolamo, 1996).

According to the DSM-IV-TR (American Psychiatric Association, 2000), risk factors for developing PTSD involve the severity, duration, and proximity of an individual's exposure to the traumatic event (Kessler et al., 1999). However, there is evidence that social supports, family history, childhood experiences, personality variables, and pre-existing mental disorders may significantly influence the development of PTSD. The DSM-IV-TR does note, however, that PTSD can develop in individuals without any predisposing conditions, particularly if the stressor is especially extreme (Dietrich, 2001). The problem with determining the extent to which individuals who have experienced prior traumatization are susceptible to developing PTSD when experiencing later events is that most research is event-specific and cannot be generalized to include all traumatic events (Dietrich, 2001). For example, the National Comorbidity Survey (Kessler et al., 1999) found that the risk of PTSD is highest for those male and female respondents who report rape, childhood physical abuse, and childhood neglect when experiencing a subsequent trauma, but the nature of the second event must also be extreme. Gender may not constitute a direct risk factor, but it may function to increase the risk of exposure to certain traumatic events such as rape (Kessler et al., 1999). Factors proposed as playing a role in the development of PTSD following exposure are described in Table 3-2.

TABLE 3-2
FACTORS PROPOSED AS PLAYING A ROLE IN THE DEVELOPMENT OF POSTTRAUMATIC STRESS DISORDER

1. Prior histories of other DSM disorders and gender (Kessler et al., 1999).
2. Genetic factors (McEwen, 2000; True & Lyons, 1999; True, Rice, Eisen, Heath, Goldberg, Lyons, & Nowak, 1993).
3. Family members who have PTSD or mood or anxiety disorders (Yehuda, 1999b).
4. Prior traumatization (particularly childhood sexual or physical abuse) (Shalev, 1996).
5. Child separation from parents
6. Family instability.
7. Predisposing mental health condition (anxiety or depression).
8. Neurocognitive factors (Orr & Pitman, 1999).
9. Impaired affect regulation or self-capacities (Briere, 2002).
10. Personality factors (Schnurr & Vielhauer, 1999) and childhood maltreatment (Briere, 2002; Nijenhuis, van der Hart, & Kruger, 2002).

Of interest, PTSD risk may be mediated by physiological sequelae following childhood maltreatment (Glaser, 2000; Ito, Teicher, Glod, Harper, Magnus, & Gelbard, 1993; Ito, Teicher, Glod, & Ackerman, 1998; Putnam & Trickett, 1997; Teicher, Glod, Surrey, & Swett, 1993). That is, it results in physiological changes that may increase the risk of exposure to traumatic stressors and/or the development of PTSD in response to subsequent stressors. It is hypothesized that persons who have experienced previous trauma(s) are at risk for developing PTSD because repeated exposure to trauma causes hyperactive release of stress hormones which may be instrumental in creating symptoms of PTSD.

Less supported in the research but of interest are three additional factors that also reflect changes in trends in protective service employment

(Norris et al., 2001). One issue is the increased presence of women in occupations once considered too dangerous for them. Even though women are still prevented by policy from serving in direct combat positions in the U.S. military, they have always been "under fire" in support roles. Minorities, those from lower socioeconomic levels, and individuals raised in traumatic and dangerous communities are also now finding employment in these field since discriminatory barriers relating to personal history have been eliminated. It is therefore relevant to consider how gender, socioeconomic status, minority status, and childhood living conditions relate to traumatic stress risk. However, it is important to caution that the data cannot be generalized to support the notion that these factors are predictive of later PTSD.

Norris et al. (2001) reported that in 42 of 45 studies, gender influenced postdisaster outcomes (93%); women or girls were affected more adversely by disasters than were men or boys. Furthermore, psychological effects were both stronger and more lasting among females. The effects occurred across a broad range of outcomes, but the strongest effects were for PTSD, for which women's rates often exceeded men's by a ratio of 2:1. Socioeconomic status (SES), as manifested by education, income, literacy, or occupational prestige, was found to affect outcomes significantly in 11 samples of disaster victims. In 10 (91%) of these, lower SES was consistently associated with greater postdisaster distress. The effect of SES increased as the severity of exposure increased. Other factors included living in a highly disrupted or traumatized community and experiencing secondary stress and resource loss. Predisaster functioning and personality influenced outcomes in 22 studies. Having a "neurotic" personality, as opposed to a stable and calm personality, increases the risk of experiencing postdisaster distress. "Hardiness" decreases this risk.

One cannot conclude, however, that an increase in women, minorities, and those with family histories of lower socioeconomic status or which a childhood spent in dangerous or violent communities accounts for the PTSD found among protective service workers today. In fact, one problem with generalizing much of the risk factor literature to protective services is the lack of data on such conditions as childhood trauma experience, lifetime trauma exposure, family history of instability and trauma, and genetic predisposition. It would be interesting to collect data on such biodata as lifetime trauma experiences to see if rates of childhood trauma are lower or higher than the national average. One might argue a self-selection out of a high-risk exposure occupation, but it may well be that childhood trauma exposure might in fact lead to the development of coping strategies that result in the same exemplary lifestyle that high-coping combat veterans evidenced when entering the profession in the 1970s. Using a trauma exposure checklist such as the Evaluation of Lifetime Stressors, Life Stressor Checklist – Revised, Potential Stressful Events Interview, or the Traumatic Events Screening Inventory to determine trauma history would not act to screen out candidates as being too risky by assuming predisposition, but such a checklist could be an indicator of high function given clean background checks coupled with trauma history. Any indication that a candidate has managed to avoid the types of behaviors and conditions that are indicative of traumatic decline, such as problems in social, occupational, and interpersonal functioning, despite early childhood and adult obstacles and traumas, suggests strong coping capability.

PERSONALITY TESTS

A much more fruitful area of exploration to find strategies to predict trauma resilience is in the use of personality tests that operationalize the competencies that contribute to hardiness or describe resiliency. An examination of the most widely used personality inventories suggests that they are not being used in this manner, although the potential exists. There is no one instrument that can be recommended to capture the attributes of stress and trauma resilience in candidates, nor is there an instrument on the market that has validity and reliability in predicting resiliency at work. Instruments under construction and validation hold promise, such as the Resilience-Builder being developed by the Center for Organizational Effectiveness (Cederholm , 2003).

At present, the most commonly used personality inventories that could be examined to determine whether factors they report could be used to operationalize competencies of stress tolerance and resilience include the following:

California Personality Inventory – CPI (Gough & Bradley, 1996) reports personality characteristics including social expertise and interpersonal style; maturity, normative orientation, and values; achievement orientation; and personal interest styles.

16PF Fifth Edition (Cattell, 1949) facilitates personnel selection and development by identifying personal qualities that influence behaviors in work settings, such as problem-solving style and inter-personal style.

NEO PI-R™ (Costa & McCrae, 1992, 1995) consists of 240 items and is considered by many psychologists to be the best inventory for mea-suring traits within the Five Factor Model (FFM) of personality.

Hogan Personality Inventory (Hogan & Hogan, 2002) is "a mea-sure of normal personality" that "evaluates the strengths and compe-tencies that enhance an individual's career; these bright side tendencies are noticed quickly by others." Available at http://www.hoganassess-ments.com/Assessments/asp

Hogan Development Survey (HDS) is "a measure of dysfunctional dispositions" that "evaluates problematic behaviors that can impede career success; these dark side behaviors appear after prolonged ac-quaintance, or during times of stress and heavy workloads." Available at http://www.hoganassessments.com/Assessments/asp

Minnesota Multiphasic Personality Inventory Personality Psy-chopathology Five (PSY-5). MMPI-2 PSY-5 (Harkness, McNulty, & benPorath, 1995) is composed of a set of scales designed to measure di-mensions of personality disorders but overlaps with the Neo-PI-R and other scales.

Taylor-Johnson Temperament Analysis (T-JTA) (Taylor & Mor-rison, 1990) is an assessment that measures personality traits that affect an individual's personal and interpersonal adjustment.

A comparison between these personality factors and those measured by other tests can be found on the IPIP website, http://ipip.ori.org (Goldberg, 1999ab), providing a sense of the personality dimension conceptualized by the individual author. Decisions about personality tests for selection/promotion should include consideration of desired competencies in personality characteristics. Determination of validity should be based on an understanding of the types of variables measured by the various tests. The instrument that captures the most important as well as the greatest number of personality variables desired in the candidate should determine final selection.

SCREENING FOR RESILIENCE

Ever since the research of Kobasa, Maddi, and Kahn (1982) on hardi-ness as a concept explaining why some people are more stress-tolerant than others, an instrument that is predictive of resilience in employees has been sought. The Hardiness Scale (Kobasa et al., 1982) included three components: commitment, challenge, and control. High levels of commitment, seeking challenge, and feelings of self-control were thought to mean high hardiness. Mental health clinicians/practitioners are being asked to develop skills to serve as management consultants to assist administrators in selecting stress/trauma hardy individuals. At the minimum, they are being asked to determine training needs that will instill resiliency in their at-risk employees (Wolin & Wolin, 1993). This approach shifts from the clinical arena; it asks employees what they are thinking rather what they are feeling. Reivich and Shatte (2002) argue that feelings are a result of thinking; therefore, by changing the way one thinks, one can control one's emotional reactions to stressful situations. They promote an "ABC" system: "A" stands for adversity (what pushes your buttons); "B" is your inherent belief about life, which triggers responding actions and feelings; and "C" is the consequences. They argue that although adversity will continue to affect us, if we analyze and revamp our beliefs, our consequences will improve, resulting in improved quality of life. Resilience assessment tools include those developed by Reivich and Shatte and and marketed by Adaptiv Systems and the Hay Group. They are the Adaptiv Resilience Factor Inventory and the RQ-60 Resilience Measure. The latter was developed for the corporate market. It rates individuals on resilience and is scored for each of 7 resilience factors and an overall resilience quotient (RQ). The seven resiliency factors used in the RFI and the RQ-60 are described in Table 3-3.

TABLE 3-3
THE SEVEN RESILIENCY FACTORS USED
IN THE RFI AND THE RQ-60

1. Emotion regulation	5. Empathy
2. Causal analysis	6. Self-efficacy
3. Impulse control	7. Reaching out
4. Optimism	

The Resiliency Map (Orioli, 2001) explores resiliency demands, assets, and current levels of functioning. The Resiliency Map contains twenty-one resiliency factor scales, and it has six separate parts. These are described in Table 3-4.

TABLE 3-4
THE RESILIENCY MAP

1. Environmental demands	Looks at the changes, pressures, and stressors that are part of everyday work, personal life, and family life.
2. Environmental assets	Determines areas of satisfaction, benefit, and support within both work and nonwork settings.
3. Resilient beliefs and values	Measures four thinking and feeling patterns that help or hinder ability to build resilience.
4. Personal coping capabilities	Explores five basic competencies that help bolster resiliency and manage demands.
5. Social coping capabilities	Covers three major areas of interpersonal support and connection.
6. Health and functioning	Describes the degree to which one is free from physical, behavioral, or emotional symptoms that reflect chronic difficulty in managing life and work demands.

SCREENING FOR EMOTIONAL INTELLIGENCE

Emotional intelligence describes a set of noncognitive skills that individuals use to cope with daily demands, pressures, other people, and themselves. According to Goleman (1997) it comprises five essential competencies; three involve how we relate to ourselves (self-awareness, regulation, and motivation), and two involve how we relate to others (empathy and effective relationships). Emotional intelligence allows us to relate to ourselves so that we can have insight into and regulate our thinking, feelings, and behavior. Relating to others is important in how we use the empathy of social support offered by others. There are four statistically reliable instruments that purport to measure emotional intelligence.

The Emotional Competency Inventory (ECI) (Boyatzis & Goleman, 1999) presents three clusters of twenty competencies of emotional intelligence. Efforts to develop a construct and criterion-related test have led to two popular tests that measure emotional intelligence. One test is the BarOn EQ-I (BarOn & Parker, 2002), which consists of 133 items and gives an overall EQ score as well as scores on five composite scales and fifteen subscales (Table 3-5).

TABLE 3-5
THE BARON EQ-I

Composite Scales	Subscales
1. Intrapersonal scales	Self-regard Emotional self-awareness Assertiveness Independence Self-actualization
2. Interpersonal scales	Empathy Social responsibility Interpersonal relationship
3. Adaptability scales	Reality testing Flexibility Problem solving
4. Stress management scales	Stress tolerance Impulse control
5. General mood scales	Optimism Happiness

The second test is the Mayer-Salovey-Caruso Emotional Intelligence Test (MSCEIT™). The MSCEIT was designed to measure the four branches of the emotional intelligence ability model of Mayer and Salovey (1997). The MSCEIT is an ability-based scale that measures how well people perform tasks and solve emotional problems, as opposed to a scale that relies on a subjective assessment of their perceived emotional skills (Salovey & Barrett, 2002). Responses to MSCEIT represent actual abilities at solving emotional problems. According to Mayer, Salovey, and Caruso (1997), this means that scores are relatively unaffected by self-concept, response set, emotional state, and other confounding conditions.

While Schnurr and Vielhauer (1999) informatively summarize personality factors that appear to present risk factors for developing PTSD, and while the vocabulary appears to overlap with the instruments presented above, it is wise to reiterate that no resiliency, hardiness, or emotional intelligence test has achieved construct and criterion related validity in predicting job performance, much less stress and traumatization on the job affecting performance. It is important to note, however, that research is well underway. In the interim, consumers of psychological tests for determining the best candidates for high-risk trauma exposure occupations should use them as descriptive, not predictive, indicators of applicants (McFarlane, 1999; Shalev, 1999; van der Kolk, McFarlane, & Weisaeth, 1996).

CONCLUSION

Psychological and personality testing is a powerful mechanism for screening potential candidates for consideration for employment in the high-risk, high-exposure occupations of the protective services and emergency medical care. Just as employers owe a duty to employees and the public to ensure the physical and medical safety of workers and those whom they serve, so too can risk-management programs be implemented in areas of human resource management other than reactive counseling. Those in the professions noted have increased their implementation of stress inoculation training as a mechanism to prepare workers for operating under violent, dangerous, and traumatic conditions. It is time to consider how administration might reduce the risk of negligent hiring by screening out those prone to stress and mental injuries such as PTSD from work events. Death, disability, injury, illness, retention, and performance data may well be improved by ensuring that the best possible, hardy worker is selected for the job.

REFERENCES

American Psychiatric Association (2000). *Diagnostic and Statistical Manual of Mental Disorders* (4th ed., text revision). Washington, DC: APA.

Bar On, R., & Parker, J. (2002). *The Handbook of Emotional Intelligence: Theory, Development, Assessment, and Application at Home, School and in the Workplace.* San Francisco, CA: Jossey-Bass.

Barrick, M., & Mount, M. (1991). The Big-Five personality dimensions and job performance: A meta-analysis. *Personnel Psychology, 44*(1), 1–26.

Block, J. (1995). Going beyond the five factors given: Rejoinder to Costa and McCrae and to Goldberg and Saucier. *Psychological Bulletin, 117,* 226–229.

Boyatzis, R. E., Goleman, D., & Hay/McBer. (1999). *Emotional Competence Inventory.* Boston: Hay/McBer Group.

Briere, J. (2002). Treating adult survivors of severe childhood abuse and neglect: Further development of an integrative model. In J. Briere, J. E. B. Myers, L. Berliner, C. T. Hendrix, C. Jenny, & T. Reid (Eds.), *The APSAC Handbook on Child Maltreatment* (2nd ed.). Available online http://www.johnbriere.com/STM.pdf, pp. 1–26). Newbury Park, CA: Sage Publications.

Cattell, R. B. (1949). Personality tests and measurements. In Delphian Society, *Patterns for Modern Living* (pp. 283–327). Chicago: Delphian Society.

Cederholm, R. (2003). *The Resiliency-Builder.* Madison, WI: Center for Organizational Effectiveness.

Costa, P. T., Jr., & McCrae, R. R. (1992). Normal personality assessment in clinical practice: The NEO Personality Inventory. *Psychological Assessment, 4,* 5–13.

Costa, P. T., Jr., & McCrae, R. R. (1995). Domains and facets: Hierarchical personality assessment using the Revised NEO Personality Inventory. *Personnel Assessment, 64,* 21–50.

Costa, P. T., Jr., McCrae, R. R., & Kay, G. G. (1995). Persons, places, and personality: Career assessment using the Revised NEO Personality Inventory. *Journal of Career Assessment, 3,* 123–139.

Davidson, J. R. T., & Foa, E. B. (1991). Diagnostic issues in posttraumatic stress disorder: Considerations for the DSM-IV. *Journal of Abnormal Psychology, 100*(3), 346–355.

Dietrich, A. M. (2001). Risk factors in PTSD and related disorders: Theoretical, treatment, and research implications [Electronic version]. *Traumatology, 7*(1). Available online http://www.fsu.edu/~trauma/v7/Riskfactorsfinal.htm.

Digman, J. (1990). Personality structure: Emergence of the five-factor model. *Annual Review of Psychology, 41,* 417–440.

Eysenck, H. J. (1991). Dimensions of personality: 16, 5 or 3? Criteria for a taxonomic paradigm. *Personality and Individual Differences, 12,* 773–90.

Glaser, D. (2000). Child abuse and neglect and the brain – A review. *Journal of Child Psychology and Psychiatry, 41*(1), 97–116.

Goldberg, L. R. (1993). The structure of phenotypic personality traits. American Psychologist, 48, 26-34.

Goldberg, L. R. (1994). How not to whip a straw dog. *Psychological Inquiry, 5*(2), 128–130.

Goldberg, L. R. (1999a). A broad-bandwidth, public-domain, personality inventory measuring the lower-level facets of several five-factor models. In I. Mervielde, I. Deary, F. De Fruyt, & F. Ostendorf (Eds.), *Personality Psychology in Europe* (Vol. 7, pp. 7–28). Tilburg, Netherlands: Tilburg University Press.

Goldberg, L. R. (1999b). The curious experiences survey, a revised version of the Dissociative Experiences Scale: Factor structure, reliability, and relations to demographic and personality variables. *Psychological Assessment, 11,* 134–145.

Goleman, D. (1997). *Emotional Intelligence.* New York: Bantam Books.

Gough, H. G., & Bradley, P. (1996). *CPI Manual* (3rd ed.). Palo Alto, CA: Consulting Psychologists Press.

Harkness, A. R., McNulty, J. L., & benPorath, Y. S. (1995). *Minnesota Multiphasic Personality Inventory Personality Psychopathology Five PSY-5.* Minneapolis, MN: University of Minnesota Press.

Hogan, R., & Hogan, J. (2002). The Hogan Personality Inventory. In B. de Raad & M. Perugini (Eds.), *Big Five Assessment* (pp. 329-351). Göttingen, Germany: Hogrefe & Huber.

Hurtz, G. M., & Donovan, J. J. (2000). Personality and job performance: The Big Five revisited. *Journal of Applied Psychology, 85,* 869–879.

International Association of Chiefs of Police (1973). *National Advisory Commission on Criminal Justice Standards and Goals: Police.* Washington, DC: U.S. Government.

Ito, Y., Teicher, M. H., Glod, C. A., & Ackerman, E. (1998). Preliminary evidence for aberrant cortical development in abused children: A quantitative EEG study. *Journal of Neuropsychiatry and Clinical Neurosciences, 10,* 298–307.

Ito, Y., Teicher, M. H., Glod, C. A., Harper, D., Magnus, E., & Gelbard, H. A. (1993). Increased prevalence of electrophysiological abnormalities in children with psychological, physical, and sexual abuse. *Journal of Neuropsychiatry and Clinical Neurosciences, 5,* 401–408.

Kessler, R. C., Sonnega, A., Bromet, E., Hughes, M., Nelson, C. B., & Breslau, N. (1999). Epidemiological risk factors for trauma and PTSD. In R. Yehuda (Ed.), *Risk Factors for Posttraumatic Stress Disorder* (pp. 23–60). Washington, DC: American Psychiatric Press.

Kobasa, S. C., Maddi, S. R., & Kahn, S. (1982). Hardiness and health: A prospective study. *Journal of Personality and Social Psychology 42,* 168–177.

Martin, I. (1996). *From Couch to Corporation: Becoming a Successful Corporate Therapist.* New York: John Wiley & Sons.

Mayer, J. D., & Salovey, P. (1997). What is emotional intelligence? In P. Salovey & D. Sluyter (Eds.), *Emotional Development and Emotional Intelligence: Implications for Educators* (pp. 3–31). New York: Basic Books.

Mayer, J. D., Salovey, P., & Caruso, D. (1997). Emotional IQ test (CD ROM). Needham, MA: Virtual Knowledge.

McCrae, R., & John, O. (1992). An introduction to the five-factor model and its applications. *Journal of Personality, 60*(2) 174–215.

McEwen, B. S. (2000). Allostasis and allostatic load: Implications for neuropsychopharmacology. *Neuropsychopharmacology, 22*(2), 108–124

McFarlane, A. C. (1999). Risk factors for the acute biological and psychological response to trauma. In R. Yehuda (Ed.), *Risk Factors for Posttraumatic Stress Disorder* (pp. 163-190). Washington, DC: American Psychiatric Press.

McFarlane, A. C., & de Girolamo, G. (1996). The nature of traumatic stressors and the epidemiology of posttraumatic reactions. In B. A. van der Kolk, A. C. McFarlane, & L. Weisaeth (Eds.), *Traumatic Stress: The Effects of Overwhelming Experience on Mind, Body, and Society* (pp. 129–154). New York: The Guilford Press.

Mount, M. K., & Barrick, M. R. (1995). The Big Five personality dimensions: Implications for research and practice in human resource management. *Research in Personnel and Human Resources Management, 13,* 153–200.

Nijenhuis, E. R. S., Van der Hart, O., & Kruger, K. (2002). The psychometric characteristics of the Traumatic Experiences Questionnaire (TEC): First findings among psychiatric outpatients. *Clinical Psychology and Psychotherapy, 9*(3), 200–210.

Norris, F. H., Byrne, C. M., Diaz, E., & Kaniasty, K. (2001). Psychosocial resources in the aftermath of natural and human-caused disasters: A review of the empirical literature, with implications for intervention. National Center for PTSD. Retrieved online October 22, 2001, at http://www.ncptsd.org/facts/disasters/fs_resources.html

Nowack, K. M. (1990). Initial development and validation of a stress and health risk factor instrument. *American Journal of Health Promotion, 4,* 173–180.

Orioli, E. (2001). EQMap. New York ESSI Systems.

Orr, S. P., & Pitman, R. K. (1999). Neurocognitive risk factors for PTSD. In R. Yehuda (Ed.), *Risk Factors for Posttraumatic Stress Disorder* (pp. 125–142). Washington, DC: American Psychiatric Press.

Paunonen, S. V., & Ashton, M. C. (2001). Big Five factors and facets and the prediction of behavior. *Journal of Personality and Social Psychology, 81,* 524–539.

Putnam, F. W., & Trickett, P. K. (1997). Psychobiological effects of sexual abuse: A longitudinal study. *Annals of the New York Academy of Sciences, 821,* 150–159.

Reivich, K., & Shatte, A. (2002). *The Resilience Factor: Seven Essential Skills for Overcoming Life's Inevitable Obstacles.* New York Broadway Books.

Salgado, J. F. (1997). The five factor model of personality and job performance in the European community. *Journal of Applied Psychology, 82,* 30–43.

Salovey, P., & Barrett, L. (2002). *The Wisdom in Feeling: Psychological Processes in Emotional Intelligence.* New York: The Guilford Press.

Schnurr, P. P., & Vielhauer, J. J. (1999). Personality as a risk factor for PTSD. In R. Yehuda (Ed.), *Risk Factors for Posttraumatic Stress Disorder* (pp. 191–222). Washington, DC: American Psychiatric Press.

Shalev, A. Y. (1996). Stress versus traumatic stress: From acute homeostatic reactions to chronic psychopathology. In B. A. van der Kolk, A. C. McFarlane, & L. Weisaeth (Eds.), *Traumatic Stress. The Effects of Overwhelming Experience on Mind, Body, and Society* (pp. 77–101). New York: The Guilford Press.

Shalev, A. Y. (1999). Psychophysiological expression of risk factors for PTSD. In R. Yehuda (Ed.), *Risk Factors for Posttraumatic Stress Disorder* (pp. 143–162). Washington, DC: American Psychiatric Press.

Slivinski, L., Loremore, A., & Miles, J. (1997). *The Wholistic Competency Profile: A Model.* Ottowa, Canada: Public Service Commission of Canada.

Taylor, R., & Morrison, L. (1990). *Taylor-Johnson Temperament Analysis.* Thousand Oaks, CA: Psychological Publications.

Teicher, M. H., Glod, C. A., Surrey, I., & Swett, C. (1993). Early childhood abuse and limbic system ratings in adult psychiatric outpatients. *Journal of Neuropsychiatry and Clinical Neurosciences, 5,* 301–306.

Territo, L., Swanson, C., & Chamelin, N. (1977). *The Police Personnel Selection Process.* Indianapolis, IN: Bobbs-Merrill.

Trull, T. J., Useda, J. D., Costa, P. T., Jr., & McCrae, R. R. (1995). Comparison of the MMPI-2 Personality Psychopathology Five (PSY-5), the NEO-PI, and NEO-PI-R. *Psychological Assessment, 7*(4), 508–516.

True, W. R., & Lyons, M. J. (1999). Genetic risk factors for PTSD: A twin study. In R. Yehuda (Ed.), *Risk Factors for Posttraumatic Stress Disorder* (pp. 61–78). Washington, DC: American Psychiatric Press.

True, W. R., Rice, J., Eisen, S. A., Heath, A. C., Goldberg, J., Lyons, M. J., & Nowak, J. (1993). A twin study of genetic and environmental contributions to liability for posttraumatic stress symptoms. *Archives of General Psychiatry, 50,* 257–264.

van der Kolk, B. A., McFarlane, A. C., & Weisaeth, L. (Eds.). (1996). Traumatic stress. *The Effects of Overwhelming Experience on Mind, Body, and Society.* New York: The Guilford Press.

Wolin, S., & Wolin, S. (1993). *The Resilient Self.* New York, NY: Villiard Books.

Yehuda, R. (1999a). *Risk Factors for Posttraumatic Stress Disorder.* Washington, DC: American Psychiatric Press.

Yehuda, R. (1999b). Parental PTSD as a risk factor for PTSD. In R. Yehuda (Ed.), *Risk Factors for Posttraumatic Stress Disorder* (pp. 93–123). Washington, DC: American Psychiatric Press.

Chapter 4

MEASURING PROTECTIVE BEHAVIORS FOR PERCEIVED RISKS OF HAZARDS

Leigh M. Smith

INTRODUCTION

When experts and members of the general public discuss hazards and risks in the context of disasters they often talk at cross-purposes. For experts (actuaries, insurance brokers, epidemiologists, and the like) assessments are made from a technical/instrumental perspective, while for the rest of us affective and personal issues imbedded in a social context of mores and values influence our judgments. Of course, the adoption of an expert perspective is not value-free. The point here is the domain of relevance and how it is constituted.

A great deal has been written about how people (lay and expert) form their judgments and how these judgments relate to actions in the face of perceived risks. This chapter is concerned with how the presence of a hazard relates to actions, in particular protective behaviors, and how the standard paradigm for measuring these behaviors fails to capture important dimensions that should prove useful in understanding their adoption.

In the technical literature a "hazard" is the precondition for a "risk," which is the cost/benefit of an event weighted by the probability of its occurrence: "cost" being reckoned in deaths and dollars. For members of the lay public costs are more broadly reckoned: psychological, economic, and social effects on self and others. Rushefsky (1982) has argued that even among experts different epistemological perspectives lead to disagreements over risks. The broader construal of costs outside expert circles is a central factor in the dissonance between the goal of risk-reduction strategies and the actions of individuals. The contention that people will change their behavior if they "know the facts" ignores the role of other personal and social factors in formation of peoples' action strategies. Too often this misplaced faith in the efficacy of "facts" in behavioral change has formed the basis of unsuccessful attempts to have communities, organizations, and individuals adopt protective behaviors and strategies against the potential negative outcomes of hazards. Facts outside their interpretive context may mean very little to the nonexpert. Subtle technical nuances do not make grist for the mills of public decision-making and action.

THE PSYCHOMETRIC APPROACH AND ITS WEAKNESSES

Although efforts to establish objective indices of risk in terms of economic and environmental damage are both necessary and valuable for planning responses to potential disasters, the emphasis in this chapter is on the psychological and behavioral responses of people to perceived dangers and their risks. The psychometric approach to risk assessment is exemplified in the work of Fischhoff, Slovic and their colleagues (Fischhoff, Lichtenstein, Slovic, Derby, & Keeney, 1981; Slovic, 1992; Slovic, Fischhoff, & Lichtenstein, 1986). Their work has been influential for theories about the factors that affect peoples' judgments of risks and how these judgments relate to the actions of individuals in relation to hazards and risks. From their own exploratory studies and findings in the literature these authors developed scales upon which risks could be evaluated. Subsequently, they went on to explore the factorial structure of the scales with a view to abstracting the major dimensions of subjective risk evaluation. They also developed a descriptive taxonomy of hazards by using a common set of scales to rate a broad range of hazards. Other authors, such as Otway and von Winterfeldt (1992), have extended the list of rating criteria while debates have proceeded in the literature over the commensurability and ubiquity of these rating criteria. However, Kraus and Slovic (1988) observed, "The dimensions of any hazard space [that is, the factor analysis of the 9 scales used by Fischhoff, Slovic, and their colleagues] are likely to be dependent on the nature of the set of hazards described" (p. 454).

The psychometric approach can be criticized on the grounds that although theorists acknowledge to some degree the social and cultural context in which the judgments are made, their linear single-level models do not adequately incorporate these influences. Kasperson, Renn, Slovic, Brown, Emel, Globe, et al. (1988), who worked within the psychometric paradigm, have written of how the perceived magnitude of risks can be affected by social process and how small actuarial risks can be perceived as far greater than their real potential. Outside this paradigm, Dake (1992) has argued that risk is socially constructed and is influenced by cultural biases and worldviews. Later, Slovic and coworkers came to the view that the way in which risks are assessed is affected by a person's worldview and emotions. They argued that worldview orients people in interpreting the exigencies of life and ordering their priorities (Slovic, Fischhoff, & Lichtenstein, 2000). While people who differ in respect of these factors may perceive a common set of risks, their rankings of the attendant dangers will vary as a function of their biases and worldviews. This process can also involve the linking of events whose values are determined by social and group norms and, consequently, through the chaining of risks, magnify or attenuate the perceived risk of the source hazard.

Notwithstanding this shift in perspective, Joffe (2003) has questioned the theoretical adequacy of the psychometric approach to an understanding of how people assess risks. For Joffe the problem lies in the metaphor of *the person as an information processing machine*, where inputs in the form of perceptions are weighted and concatenated to form a judgment. Joffe sees two problems with this approach. First, it does not explain how and why people make the judgments they make. Second, it is based on the assumption that all or most of what is relevant to the way people act in the face of a potential hazard is determined by individual consciousness. It is Joffe's view that "individuals faced with potential danger operate from a position of anxiety that motivates them to represent the danger in a specific way" (p. 62). Social Representation Theory (Flick, 1998; Moscovici, 1998; Moscovici & Duveen, 2001) provides a framework for describing the process whereby a person anchors and objectifies common sense (including the lay apprehension of risk). Anchoring involves the use of familiar symbols and metaphors to make sense of the potential risk. The repertoire of metaphors, which Joffe (2003) describes as the "trove of familiarity" (p. 64), is both constructed and employed in the public domain by such processes as the transformation of scientific discourse into media reportage. Objectification works in conjunction with anchoring by aligning the particularities of the current risk with the metaphorical attributes of the past event to which it is being linked. It is not unreasonable to posit these processes also result from formal and informal organizational cultures.

With similar concerns, Shinn and Toohey (2003) have identified a failure in conceptualization that they call the *context minimisation error.* This error consists in not taking into account the context in which a person makes decisions about change. The studies they review provide evidence for community-level factors, which are not apprehended consciously, that affect people's judgments and behaviors. Shinn and Toohey show how such factors can moderate the relations among individual-level factors. It follows that in attempting to change people's protective behaviors, those responsible need to bring about social and organizational changes as well as individual changes because the meaning of the behaviors has to become embedded at the organizational level.

Waring and Glendon (1998) have provided an overview of the processes involved in risk cognition, including a matrix of the decision-making and action-trajectory of individual behavior in the face of danger. However, the existence of supraindividual influences on individual decision-making in respect to hazards suggests that any attempt to incorporate psychometric measures into individual-level models of the belief-behavior link will fail to the extent that supraindividual processes are relevant and uncaptured in individual ratings. The segmentation of the analyses of risks through a typology of hazards cannot adequately cope with the problem because it fails to capture the social and cultural influences that drive respondents' judgments. Elsewhere (Smith & Violanti, 2003), I have recommended the use of multilevel models for unraveling the relation between risk perceptions, the mediators of the effects, and the outcomes of being exposed to hazards. A schematic multilevel model for the adoption of protective behaviors is shown in Figure 4.1. The components of the categories of influence are not detailed; however, a description and rationale for the individual-level and community-level factors are given in Smith and Violanti (2003).

A BETTER APPROACH TO MEASUREMENT

In studying human behavior, researchers are typically interested in the internal psychological causes (traits, beliefs, attitudes, moods, motives,

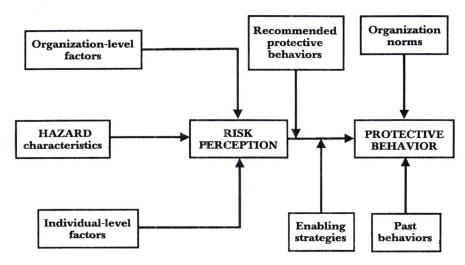

Figure 4-1. A multilevel model for the adoption of protective behaviors.

and intentions) of the actors' behaviors and the effects of past behaviors on present behaviors. In the field of disaster research the behaviors that are the focus include current reactions to disaster situations (past and/or present) and the way in which previous behavior, training, and experience affect adaptation and reaction to disasters. This includes such reactions as those classified as *protective behaviors* (van der Plight, 1996; Weinstein, 1989; Weinstein, Lyon, Rothman, & Cuite, 2000; Windle, 1999). The problem for the researcher is how to assess behaviors in a manner that facilitates modeling their role in the adaptation/reaction process. In short, how are they adequately measured? In what follows, I suggest why using the factor-analytic measurement paradigm for traits, attitudes, and the like is not appropriate and outline an approach to measurement that takes better account of the nature of inventories of behaviors.

For many psychological constructs measurement consists in having the person respond to a set of questions chosen to directly reflect the construct. Self-report attitude and belief scales take this form. Other measures, as in the case of personality traits, are of a similar format; however, the relation between the items in the questionnaire and the traits may be less transparent. The items for these scales might not obviously look like they relate to the construct (have face validity). Where psychological constructs are assessed by ratings, the measure of the construct is determined as a weighted sum of the item ratings (e.g., estimated factor scores), the weights having been determined on the basis of a previously established theoretically motivated analysis of a normative sample. Such analyses are generally termed "normative structural analyses" and typically use data analytic techniques such as factor analysis to determine the relation between constructs and items and their associated weights. This means of establishing measures, the *trait-measurement paradigm*, is more or less ubiquitous for psychological characteristics that are assessed by rating scales.

The trait-measurement paradigm posits a latent variable (Bollen, 2002) that cannot be directly observed and so must be measured indirectly using observed responses (ratings) of variables that are hypothesized to be causally linked to it. In the trait-measurement paradigm these observed variables are the items, usually in the form of statements, which constitute the scale. Such an item for a personality trait measure might read, "I enjoy being alone" and the rating required "never, infrequently, occasionally, often, always." The ratings of the items are hypothesized to be causally affected by the respondents' levels of the latent variable (trait), say introversion. The use of factor analysis to analyze this and similar data involves a commitment to the ontology of latent variables. This is not always recognized where factor analysis is used as a data reduction method for constructing a single index to represent a set of items. While principal components analysis does not carry the same ontological commitment, it is often used interchangeably for factor analysis (Gorsuch, 1990; Mulaik, 1990). Since principal components analysis is mistakenly used interchangeably with factor analysis, the arguments here regarding the trait-measurement paradigm include the use of this analytic method.

Instruments for the assessment of psychological constructs can be based upon self-ratings or ratings by other people (e.g., parents, peers, supervisors, or psychologists). They can also require respondents to perform certain structured tasks or to answer questions with fixed performance criteria (e.g., intelligence tests). Notwithstanding the form of these assessments, what all share is the assumption, crudely speaking, that people can be allocated a relative or absolute position on an index that reflects the degree to which the construct *is present in them.* The items constitute a sample of the possible manifestations of the construct that can provide a window on *a psychological entity that cannot be directly observed.*

There are, however, situations in which researchers need to shift their focus from the internal states that are the causes or effects of behaviors to the behaviors themselves. Protective behaviors are a case in point. The "measurement" of such behaviors can be problematic, especially when the paradigm for measuring internal states is applied to them. For a given situation, say an earthquake, it is possible to specify a set of behaviors that would form a useful preparation for such a contingency. A list of protective behaviors for individuals, organizations, and communities at risk for earthquake activity can be generated by analyzing what people have done in previous earthquakes and by an analysis of the attendant dangers.

In a scale for the measurement of a trait, an individual's rating of each item is hypothesized to be directly affected by the level of the trait. In practice, the ratings vary under two influences – the effect of the trait and the effect of other nontrait influences. In Classical Measurement Theory the latter are presumed to be relatively small and *random*. Thus each item is an imperfect indicator of the trait. A necessary assumption is that the items form a unidimensional set; that is, they all measure the same thing. The use of multiple items for the measurement of a trait enables an estimate of the error to be made and consequently the reliability of the measure. In the case of constructs that are less stable than traits (beliefs, moods, intentions, etc.), a change in rating by a respondent is taken as indicative of a change in their level of the construct. For rating scales of stable and varying psychological constructs, the items are considered to be a sample drawn from a hypothetical population of items that are potentially interchangeable.

The item set for a protective-behavior inventory differs in two major respects from a set of items purporting to reflect the type of construct treated as a trait. First, the protective-behavior inventory is not a sample of interchangeable indicators; it is a prescribed set of activities. It is possible that other behaviors, potentially indicative of a greater level of protection, could be added to, or substituted for, existing behaviors. This differs from adding or substituting items in a measurement scale for a trait. There, a better item more reliably reflects the trait; *it does not affect the extent to which the trait is present in the person being assessed.* Modifications of a protective-behavior inventory can result in a change of responses that do not reflect random error. There is a strong disanalogy here between the two forms of measure. Changing items in a trait scale should only lead to random variation in the ranking of individuals, whereas changing the protective-behavior inventory can lead to systematic changes in the rank order of people on the basis of their responses aggregated across the items in the inventory. A change of ranking as a consequence of the substitution of items or the addition of items in a behavior inventory may reflect real differences between the original inventory and the new inventory. Under such circumstances scores from the two scales would not be commensurable. This is undesirable and suggests that the trait-measurement paradigm is an inappropriate model for a unitary measure or index derived from a behavior inventory.

The second difference follows from the first. It has to do with the nature of the tasks and the implications these have for the type of derived measure that is appropriate for behavior inventories. It can be the case that some behaviors are hierarchically dependent on others. For example, if you do not have a torch and an earthquake leads to a total power failure at night, there may be protective behaviors you cannot initiate for want of a light. Of each behavior in an inventory we can ask: "How difficult is it to achieve?" and "How effective is it?" These two questions suggest that individuals and items (behaviors) can be ranked on the basis of these two criteria. The simultaneous ranking of items and respondents is called *conjoint measurement* (Karabatsos, 2001; Suppes, Krantz, Luce, & Tversky, 1989) and is the basis of the measurement paradigm known as *Item Response Theory* (Bond and Fox, 2001; Embretson, 1996; Embretson and Reise, 2000; Fox and Jones, 1998; Thissen and Wainer, 2001).

The problem for a researcher lies in how to use the respondents' ratings of the behaviors in the inventory. The researcher could examine the relation between each item in the inventory as a discrete variable and any other facet of the research situation. However, there is an obvious sense in which this strategy abandons the notion of the set of behaviors as possessing any collective properties. This strategy also has undesirable technical consequences such as the inflation of type I errors. Another unsatisfactory response to the problem is to aggregate the information by naively summing the ratings of the items. Because the items are not qualitatively equivalent (unlike trait items that do not differ qualitatively, only quantitatively – ex hypothesis they measure the same ontological state), two respondents can have the same sum based on different item subsets with the extreme possibility that they share no common items. A simple example would be a four-item scale (a, b, c, d) with a rating protocol (present = 1, absent = 0). Two individuals could have the same score 2 while their profiles might be quite different ("1, 1, 0, 0" and "0, 0, 1, 1"). What sense, then, can be made of the quantitatively equal scores of these two individuals? Not much, and even less of any relation such scores might have with other quantitative variables. Even where the set of behaviors has been tested for unidimensionality by factor analysis or principal components analysis it is not clear what substantive interpretation can be given to such an aggregation. Where the dimensionality of the item set is unknown, the interpretation problem is insuperable.

This problem can be overcome where items/behaviors differ in their efficacy (more or less protective) and/or difficulty to achieve. Most behavior inventories, such as protective behaviors, have one or both of these properties. Efficacy can be dealt with in several ways: actuarially, where such data exist; on the basis of expert judgment, where items are assigned weights by the experts; or through the judgments of the respondents. These considerations suggest two approaches to the construction of measures that make use of the information in the set of items as a whole.

The first approach consists in the provision of differential weights for the items. These weights could be derived from expert ratings of the efficacy of the behaviors or from empirical evidence of their protective efficacy. A second and less obvious approach is to make use of the item response data. The use of Item Response Theory (IRT) models, such as Rasch Scaling, can facilitate the development of measures with the desirable property that items form an "achievement" hierarchy. Given such a scale, individuals can be allocated locations (scores) on this hierarchy (measure) that reflect the pattern of their responding to the item set and the property of interest of the individual items that form the scale. In IRT a person's score on a measure depends on the pattern of the responses, as the items are not equally indicative of the level of the measure. Such an approach to assessing behavior inventories is manifestly preferable to the simple aggregation of responses to a list of qualitatively different items. This measurement strategy can also be used to combine respondents' ratings with the ratings of the efficacy of the behaviors derived from expert judges. These expert ratings are also amenable to IRT analysis.

In applying the IRT paradigm to the analysis of response data, we shall be concerned with two prototypical scales. The first inventory is a checklist where respondents are required to indicate whether the statement applies to them or not. The second is a set of statements that respondents are required to rate on an ordinal (Likert) protocol. Table 4-1 illustrates the first type of measurement instrument, an extract from a

TABLE 4-1
ITEMS FROM A HYPOTHETICAL PROTECTIVE BEHAVIORS CHECKLIST

	Yes	No
I have a copy of the organization's "What to do if there is a fire."		
I have read "What to do if there is a fire."		
I have attended fire drills.		
I have inspected the assembly points.		
I have practiced how to shut down my equipment in an emergency.		
Etc.		

TABLE 4-2
ITEMS FROM A HYPOTHETICAL RATING SCALE OF
WITHIN-ORGANIZATION PROTECTIVE BEHAVIORS

Rate each of these statements on the scale 1. I would never do this. 2. I would find this very difficult to do. 3. I would be able to do this. 4. I intend to do this soon. 5. I have done this in the last 12 months					
Read about fire risks	1	2	3	4	5
Undertake a CPR course	1	2	3	4	5
Bring fire risks I see to the attention of management	1	2	3	4	5
Raise issues about fire risks at staff meetings	1	2	3	4	5
Criticize current fire-emergency procedures at staff meetings	1	2	3	4	5
Discuss fire-emergency procedures with fellow workers	1	2	3	4	5
Organize a fire-safety meeting among fellow workers	1	2	3	4	5
Etc.	1	2	3	4	5

checklist of fire-emergency protective behaviors. Table 4-2 is an example of the second type of measurement instrument, an extract from a rating scale of within-organization protective behaviors.

It should be apparent that both scales contain items that are qualitatively different from each other. The first scale is a set of behaviors that have been deemed to be useful protective behaviors in the event of a fire. As argued above it does not make sense to analyze this scale as if it were a unidimensional indicator of an underlying response disposition. The behaviors are in all likelihood driven by a variety of attitudes, beliefs, personality traits, and life contingencies. The second scale also has qualitatively different items. Here the task is to indicate the difficulty in carrying out the behavior.

The data generated by the first inventory would be in the form of a string of ones and zeros for each respondent [($R_1 = 0\ 0\ 1\ 0\ 1\ 1\ 0\ \ldots$); ($R_2 = 1\ 0\ 0\ 1\ \ldots$); etc]. The simple aggregate approach would be a count of the number of items endorsed by each respondent [$R_1 = 12$; $R_2 = 9$; etc]. The problems associated with this method of generating a score from an inventory have been discussed above. The factor analytic approach (trait-measure paradigm) would examine the covariance matrix of the ratings to determine their dimensionality. A unidimensional subset of items with acceptable loadings on a single factor would then be selected to represent the "scale." Normalized factor-scores would then be calculated for each individual as their score for the scale [$R_1 = 1.2$; $R_2 = -0.8$; etc].

A closer examination of these hypothetical scores reveals that the simple aggregate only contains information about the respondent in the form of how many items he or she endorsed. This is wholly dependent upon the arbitrary list of items that forms the inventory. The factor-scores contain some information about the items. The factor-score is a reflection of something the items have in common (their unidimensionality):

$$FS_j = w_1 i_{1j} + w_2 i_{2j} + \ldots w_n i_{nj} \textbf{ (for the } j^{th} \textbf{ case on the items)}$$

These scores can be used to provide normative information on individuals in relation to the unidimensional component of the inventory. The differences between individuals cannot be interpreted as differences in magnitude — only as differences in rank. Notwithstanding this limitation, factor-scores on inventories are often used as if they are ratio measures.

The one-parameter IRT model, the Rasch model (Rasch, 1960), overcomes the limitations of simple aggregate scores and factor-scores by generating a ratio measure where differences in scores are consistent across the full range of scores. The Rasch model, where it fits the data, produces a ratio measure in the form of logit scores.[1,2] The use of the Rasch model to construct a scale involves the selection of items that can be arranged from the most endorsed to the least endorsed. Hierarchical precedence is the second property the items need to display to be included in the scale. If a person has endorsed item k, then that person should have endorsed all the preceding items. This Guttman scaling requirement (Nunnally & Bernstein, 1994) is too stringent, and a probabilistic hierarchy, as represented in Figure 4-2, is accepted.

Bond and Fox (2001) have presented a useful pictorial representation of the Rasch model as a pathway with stepping-stones. The pathway, calibrated in logits, goes from items that are easy for nearly all people to endorse, to items that are difficult to endorse. The center of each stepping-stone represents the location of an item or a person and the diameter of the stepping-stone represents the standard error of the estimate. The edges of the path mark the limits of acceptable fit for individuals and items. Figure 4-3 illustrates these points. The lighter stepping-stones depict a hypothetical outcome for the behavior checklist described above and the darker ones a selection of respondents.

There is an apparent problem in the application of the Rasch scaling model to behavior inventories. Much of this chapter has been concerned with arguing against the use of the trait-measurement paradigm as a method for combining the information in response profiles into a single variable score. The argument centers on the point that the items are typically not indices of a single underlying generative mechanism or trait. The Rasch model also assumes that the items form a unidimensional set. The issue is whether or not the meaning of "unidimensional" is commensurate with its use in factor analysis as it is applied in the trait-measurement paradigm. If it is commensurate, then presumably the same objections apply.

Factor analysis has its origins in an ontological question about the nature of intelligence, namely, whether all manifestations of intelligence have their genesis in a single cause. This is not the place to debate questions about the nature of intelligence. My purpose is to point out that the factor analysis model assumes that there are underlying psychological

---

[1] Logit = natural logarithm of the odds ratio; namely, in [(probability of endorsing item) / (1 – probability of endorsing item)].

[2] In general, technical issues will not be dealt with in this paper. Details can be found in the references. In order of difficulty, they are Bond and Fox (2001), Embretson and Reise (2000), and Thissen and Wainer (2001).

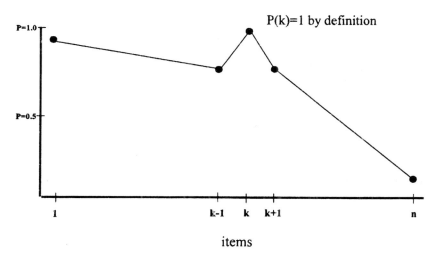

Figure 4-2. Hypothetical item response probabilities for people who endorsed item k.

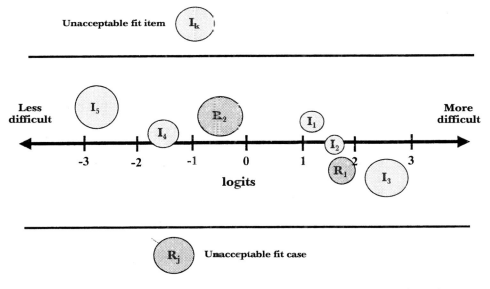

Figure 4-3. Rasch model diagram adapted from Fox and Jones (1998.)

causes that account for the covariation of the events that we observe and that covariation of peoples' responses conform to the Classical Measurement Model.[3] Some users of factor analysis understand it instrumentally

---

[3] Later factor analytic models allow for different measurement models (such as correlated errors); however, this does not affect the thrust of the argument presented here.

as a method of data reduction. However, data reduction is more consistent with principal components analysis. The difference between factor analysis and principal components analysis lies in how error is modeled. Where the results of a principal component analysis are interpreted as underlying causal mechanisms, that is where the components are interpreted as things (states, traits, etc.), it is being used analogously to factor analysis. I have already suggested that this leads to the same disanalogy as factor analysis in the analysis of behavior inventories.

There have been several criticisms of the unreflective use of the factor analytic approach to measurement centered on the nature and direction of influences among observed variables (item responses), latent variables, and theoretical constructs (Bollen, 2002; Bollen & Lennox, 1991; Edwards & Bagozzi, 2000). The key issues are as follows:

1. If a construct is conceptualized as a latent variable, is it a cause[4] or effect of the observed variable(s)?

2. Are the influences between variables (latent and observed, observed and observed, latent and latent) direct or indirect?

3. Are the observed variables modeled with or without error components?

These authors argue that an analysis of the means for deriving a measure of a construct must address the three issues. Bollen and Lennox (1991) have shown how the inappropriate use of a measurement model that assumes that responses to observed variables are caused by a latent variable (an effect indicator model) leads to incorrect predictions about how the observed variables should covary and consequently to false expectations about item consistency and the reliability of the composite measure. In addition, Edwards and Bagozzi (2000) have provided a taxonomy of relationships among indicators and latent variables together with guidelines for deciding which model is most appropriate for a given measurement situation. In some respects, the points these authors make are consistent with the concerns expressed here about the use of the trait-measurement paradigm for deriving composite measures of sets of heterogeneous items. However, there is an important additional concern addressed here: The hierarchical ordering of items.

The meaning of "unidimensional" in the Rasch model differs from the meaning in factor analysis. Like factor analysis the Rasch model was

---

[4] Rather than adopt a particular conception of causality, Edwards and Bagozzi (2000) opt for the less philosophically loaded notion of influence. Discussions about cause in this chapter should be understood in this broad sense.

first applied to the measurement of abilities. The analytic model is based on the assumptions that a criterion of success can be set for each item and that performance on the items (manifestations of the ability) can be ordered in terms of difficulty. The key to unidimensionality here is whether the items (say questions in a test of mathematical ability) can be ordered in difficulty such that the orderings are consistent across respondents. Items that do not meet this criterion are eliminated. A set of items that meet the criterion when the Rasch model is applied are said to be unidimensional. It should be clear that this notion of unidimensionality differs from the use of the term in factor analysis and the trait-measurement paradigm. It also needs to be recognized that it is possible for a set of items to be unidimensional in both senses.

The important difference lies in the possibility of a set of items to be Rasch (1960) unidimensional but not factor analysis unidimensional, even if the use of a factor analysis program appears to indicate a single factor. There are insufficient constraints in the factor analysis model to distinguish between a unidimensional matrix of contingent covariances and a unidimensional matrix of covariances driven by a single mechanism. The Rasch model informs us about both the respondents *and* the items. The ranking reflects the difficulty respondents have endorsing the items. How, then, do difficulty hierarchies arise?

The ability hierarchy is the paradigm structure for the Rasch model. The two facets of this structure are items that differ in difficulty and people differing in the reference ability. The ordering of the items in terms of difficulty is just a function of ability:

$$D_1 = f \text{ (ability level reflected by each item)}$$

In the case of items from a behavior inventory, these may differ on a host of dimensions relevant to people's responses. Nonetheless, it may be possible to order the items consistently across respondents. For example the difficulty order of a set of protective behaviors may be:

$$D_2 = f \text{ (cost; availability; efficacy; ...)}$$

The facets of the D_2 function can be subject to extrinsic contingencies, such as a cost subsidy. In the ordinary course of events this is not the case with the D_1 function. It may also be the case that D_2 is specific to partitions of the respondent population based upon social and cultural factors. In other words, D_2 may be moderated by supraindividual factors that can be accommodated either as additional components of the function or by estimating separate functions based upon these extrinsic moderators.

Researchers have recognized the need to combine information about respondents' reactions to items by requiring ratings on several protocols for each item; e.g., "How often has this happened to you?" and "How stressful was it?" The responses are usually combined multiplicatively. While superficially appealing, this strategy has three problems. First, it does not overcome the objections already raised concerning trait-paradigm measures. Second, the resultant measure contains a multiplicative error component that can result in a measure with poor reliability. Third, it does not account for supraindividual influences on responses to scale items. The Rasch model is a two-facet model (ability, difficulty); however, in many situations peoples' responses are formed by more than two influences. The model has been extended by Linacre (1994) to incorporate multiple facets. The function D_2 explicitly extends the list of influences. The measure generated through the application of the multi-facet model reflects the pattern of responses across the facets, does not have the first two problems of multiplicative indices, and can potentially avoid the third.

It is an empirical question whether D_2 is consistent across respondents or segmented by social and cultural factors that influence their risk assessment of potential hazards. Where D_2 is consistent, the utility of the scores derived from the scale is also an empirical question. The scores may or may not prove useful in predicting peoples' responses to other variables and, in turn, may or may not have a role to play as proximal "causes" in a structural model. A comparison of D_1 and D_2 also highlights the point made previously that the items of a trait-like measure are interchangeable within the limits of measurement error, while the items in an inventory are qualitatively distinct.

In the concluding chapter of their book Embretson and Reise (2000) address some of the limitations of IRT models. The authors draw attention to the distinction made by Bollen and Lennox (1991) between latent variables with effect indicators and emergent variables with cause indicators. They remark that "IRT modeling is clearly a latent variable measurement model, and attempting to fit constructs that don't fit this mold is bound to lead to problems" (p. 324). It is not clear, though, that the notion of a latent variable implied in IRT is coextensive with the notion of latent variable that underwrites common factor analysis. It cannot be argued that an ordering based on difficulty is the consequence of a common cause in any unitary sense. It is more often the consequence of a variety of causes and constraints affecting how individuals develop their repertoire of protective behaviors.

CONCLUSION

Notwithstanding the case put here that the notion of "latent variable" differs between the trait-measurement paradigm and the IRT models, the question remains on the appropriateness of IRT models for behavior inventories. If, as is argued here, there is no underlying *unidimensional* cause of responses to the item set, how could the IRT model fit the data? One answer to this question is relatively trivial: The proof of the pudding is in the eating. However, this is not particularly satisfying, as I have argued this intrinsic criterion does not justify the use of factor analysis even if a one-factor model fits the data. The important question is whether the IRT model provides a better analogy for the data than the common factor analysis model. This is the nub of what has been argued here.

It is important to recognize that an IRT model can be used in two modes: for analysis of the structure of response data or as a template for the construction of a scale and its associated measure. This distinction forms something of a bone of contention in the IRT literature. This paper is not an attempt to argue the case for either position as the "proper" use of IRT. Both uses of IRT seem to be legitimate depending upon one's goal. Here the emphasis is on the construction of scales and their associated measures in a manner that suits the desirable hierarchical structure for a behavior inventory. To be explicit, I am suggesting that the utility of behavior inventories is potentially greater if they consist of an ordered set of items reflecting the "difficulty" of engaging in the behaviors as a means to a specific outcome (say, being well protected against the possible effects of an organizational disaster such as a fire). Clearly this is a restricted use of IRT; however, it is justifiable and informative for behavior inventories.

REFERENCES

Bollen, K. A. (2002). Latent variables in psychology and the social sciences. *Annual Review of Psychology, 53,* 605–634.

Bollen, K. A., & Lennox, R. (1991). Conventional wisdom on measurement: A structural equation perspective. *Psychological Bulletin, 110*(2), 305–314.

Bond, T. G., & Fox, C. M. (2001). Applying the Rasch Model: *Fundamental Measurement in the Human Sciences.* Mahwah, NJ: Lawrence Erlbaum.

Dake, K. (1992). Myths of nature and the public. *Journal of Social Issues, 48*(4), 21–38.

Edwards, J. R., & Bagozzi, R. P. (2000). On the nature and direction of relationships between constructs and measures. *Psychological Methods, 5*(2), 155–174.

Embretson, S. E. (1996). The new rules of measurement. *Psychological Assessment, 8*(4), 341–349.

Embretson, S. E., & Reise, S. P. (2000). *Item Response Theory for Psychologists.* Mahwah, NJ: Lawrence Erlbaum.

Fischhoff, B., Lichtenstein, S., Slovic, P., Derby, S. L., & Keeney, R. L. (1981). *Acceptable Risk.* Cambridge: Cambridge University Press.

Flick, U. (Ed.). (1998). *The Psychology of the Social.* Cambridge: Cambridge University Press.

Fox, C. M., & Jones, J. A. (1998). Uses of Rasch modeling in counseling psychology. *Journal of Counseling Psychology, 45*(1), 30–45.

Gorsuch, R. L. (1990). Common factor analysis versus component analysis: Some well and little known facts. *Multivariate Behavioural Research, 25*(1), 33–39.

Joffe, H. (2003). Risk: From perception to social representation. *British Journal of Social Psychology, 42,* 55–73.

Karabatsos, G. (2001). The Rasch model, additive conjoint measurement, and new models of probabilistic measurement theory. *Journal of Applied Measurement, 2*(4), 389–423.

Kasperson, R. E., Renn, O., Slovic, P., Brown, H. S., Emel, J., Globe, R., et al. (1988). The social implication of risk: A conceptual framework. *Risk Analysis, 8*(2), 177–187.

Kraus, N. N., & Slovic, P. (1988). Taxonomic analysis of perceived risk: Modeling individual and group perceptions within homogeneous hazard domains. *Risk Analysis, 8*(3), 435–455.

Linacre, J. M. (1994). Constructing measurement with a many-facet Rasch model. In M. Wilson (Ed.), *Objective measurement: Theory into Practice: Vol. 2* (pp. 129–144). Norwood, NJ: Ablex.

Moscovici, S. (1998). The history and actuality of social representation. In U. Flick (Ed.), *The Psychology of the Social* (pp. 209–247). Cambridge: Cambridge University Press.

Moscovici, S., & Duveen, G. (Eds.). (2001). *Social Representations: Explorations in Social Psychology.* Cambridge: Polity Press.

Mulaik, S. A. (1990). Blurring the distinctions between component analysis and common factor analysis. *Multivariate Behavioural Research, 25*(1), 53–59.

Nunnally, J. C., & Bernstein, I. H. (1994). *Psychometric Theory.* New York: McGraw-Hill Inc.

Otway, H., & von Winterfeldt, D. (1992). Expert judgement in risk analysis and management: Process, context and pitfalls. *Risk Analysis, 12*(1), 83–93.

Rasch, G. (1960). *Probabilistic Models for Some Intelligence and Attainment Tests.* Chicago: University of Chicago Press.

Rushefsky, M. (1982). Technical disputes Why experts disagree. *Policy Studies Review, 1*(4), 676–685.

Shinn, M., & Toohey, S. M. (2003). Community contexts of human welfare. *Annual Review of Psychology, 54,* 427–459.

Slovic, P. (1992). Perceptions of risk: Reflections on the psychometric paradigm. In S. Krimsky & D. Golding (Eds.), *Social Theories of Risk* (pp. 117–152). Westport, CT: Praeger.

Slovic, P., Fischhoff, B., & Lichtenstein, S. (1986). The psychometric study of risk perception. In V. T. Covello, J. Menkes, & J. Mumpower (Eds.), *Risk Evaluation and Management* (pp. 3–24). New York: Plenum Press.

Slovic, P., Fischhoff, B., & Lichtenstein, S. (2000). Rating the risks. In P. Slovic (Ed.), *Risk Perception* (pp. 104–120). London: Earthscan.

Smith, L. M., & Violanti, J. M. (2003). Risk response model. In D. Paton, J. M. Violanti, & L. M. Smith (Eds.), *Promoting Capabilities to Manage Posttraumatic Stress: Perspectives on Resilience* (pp. 185–203). Springfield, IL: Charles C Thomas.

Suppes, P., Krantz, D. M., Luce, R., & Tversky, A. (1989). *Foundations of Measurement.* San Diego, CA: Academic Press.

Thissen, D., & Wainer, H. (Eds.). (2001). *Test Scoring.* Mahwah, NJ: Lawrence Erlbaum.

van der Plight, J. (1996). Risk perception and self-protective behavior. *European Psychologist, 1*(1), 34–43.

Waring, A., & Glendon, A. I. (1998). *Managing Risk.* London: International Thomson Business Press.

Weinstein, N. (1989). Effects of personal experience on self-protective behavior. *Psychological Bulletin, 105*(1), 31–50

Weinstein, N., Lyon, J. E., Rothman, A. J., & Cuite, C. L. (2000). Preoccupation and affect as predictors of protective action following natural disaster. *British Journal of Health Psychology, 5*(4), 351–363.

Windle, M. (1999). Critical conceptual and measurement issues in the study of resilience. In M. D. Glantz & J. L. Johnson (Eds.), *Resilience and Development: Positive Life Adaptations. Longitudinal Research in the Social and Behavioral Sciences* (pp. 161–176). New York: Kluwer Academic/Plenum Publishers.

Chapter 5

POLICE TRAUMA: PAST EXPOSURES AND PRESENT CONSEQUENCES

STEPHANIE SAMUELS

INTRODUCTION

After working for over a decade with police officers with posttraumatic stress disorder (PTSD), three common threads have emerged. First, officers were exposed to some type of trauma or abuse (sexual, physical, emotional, or neglect) as a child. This trauma can also include significant early loss. Second, individuals who were used to being in crisis as children do very well under such conditions, but less well with "calm." Third, there often is an unresolved issue with a father figure, with a surprising number of officers having been adopted. As a consequence, many officers enter police work with PTSD and are not aware of it. Many officers come to the job numb, believing that they will not have a full career, marriage, or life span. They appear hypervigilant, have difficulty falling and staying asleep, and avoid thoughts, feelings and conversations that remind them of the event. Like many survivors, they have repressed these memories and locked them away for what they hope will be forever. My job is not only to debrief officers after critical incidents, but to open Pandora's box and return them to a higher level of functioning than they had been at prior to seeking help. This work provides the foundation for this chapter, particularly in regard to whether officers' prior traumas help or hinder them on the job. Trauma and abuse histories are not generally assessed, yet their long-term ramifications for officers' well-being and performance render them potentially important risk factors.

I am always surprised by professional police psychologists talking about the "paranoid cop." Yet, in over a decade of working with the law enforcement community, I have not met a paranoid cop. *Paranoia* is defined as "a tendency on the part of an individual or group toward excessive or irrational suspiciousness and distrustfulness of others" (American Psychiatric Association, *Diagnostic and Statistical Manual of Mental Disorders*, 1994, p. 634). "Paranoia" is not paranoia if you know what there is to be afraid of. For example, one officer that I see, Kevin, lost his brother Sergeant in a random police execution. Sergeant was ordering Chinese food when he was shot in the head from behind by a perpetrator who was running from the police in Boston and decided that he wanted to take "one of theirs" before he died. Kevin was still in the police academy and never got to fulfill his dream of working alongside his brother. One morning after a ride along with Kevin on a midnight shift, we went out to Dunkin Donuts (I wanted a cup of coffee, not him). I watched him walk into the store, go directly against the left wall, and not leave that location until I had paid and was ready to leave. This incident gave us an insight to talk about. If one could use a memory eradication device, I do not know one law enforcement officer who would not opt for it.

Herman (1992) describes how studying trauma confronts both human vulnerability in the natural world and the capacity for evil in human nature. When the events are natural disasters or "acts of God," those who bear witness sympathize readily with the victim. But when the traumatic events are of human design, those who bear witness are caught in the conflict between victim and perpetrator. It is morally impossible to remain neutral in this conflict. The bystander is forced to take sides. It is very tempting to take the side of the perpetrator. All the perpetrator asks is that the bystander do nothing. The victim, on the contrary, asks the bystander to share the burden of pain. The victim demands action, engagement, and remembering (Herman, 1992). It is my job to bear witness to the pain of these officers caught up in these circumstances and to take the action needed, talk about the incident(s), and always help them and me to remember.

The mental health community has done a tremendous disservice to our officers and the public by ignoring the glaring statistics and research. One woman in three has been sexually abused in childhood (Russell, 1984). In my practice, two out of three female officers have been sexually abused. Physical abuse occurs at about the same percentage among my male officers. There is also a higher rate of child sexual abuse among the male officers in my practice than that which is documented.

The highest suicide rates in law enforcement occur in the newer officers and not among the older ones. This finding is the opposite of national suicide statistics and may reflect older officers' military service. They came on the job with PTSD, already numb to what they would be exposed to. Younger officers without prior military service seem to have a more difficult time adjusting to the job. Prior trauma history is thus indicated. The other predetermining factor is how a person has handled a crisis in the past. The number one predictor of who will complete suicide is someone who has made a prior attempt.

Although most of the officers I see have a history of abuse, I have never seen one who is a deliberate abuser. The officers who typically end up in therapy are the ones who care, the ones who all of a sudden begin to feel and do not know why. It should be noted that I do not see mandates – officers taken off the job for whom a condition of returning to work or not being disciplined is seeing a therapist. I believe these officers, who have the same history, have become abusers and not protectors. If the history is not looked into, rehabilitation will be incomplete. One must understand one's past to liberate oneself from it and learn to do differently. My role is to provide the tools to facilitate this process. By the time that officers leave my practice, they have a plethora of tools, some they had never heard of. It is their job to build their own house; it is mine to see that they are using the right tools.

CASE STUDY: BILL

One of my first cases was an officer with 18 years of service. The officer, whom I will call "Bill," was on his normal patrol when he came up to a wooded area that should have been chained shut. Bill got out of his police car and walked up the hill to investigate further. He found himself being shot at from a distance and could not determine where the bullets were coming from. He lay on his stomach, gun drawn, prepared to return gunfire, but never had a shot because of the lack of visibility. Bill was able to crawl back down the hill and call for back-up. He stated that the shots were going just over his head. When back-up arrived and the scene was secured, it was determined that a bunch of young adults had broken into this location and were shooting target practice. The target was on the tree that turned out to be just above Bill's head. The youths had never seen the officer. While this was being sorted out, Bill was taken to hospital for chest pains and shortness of breath. He was having a panic attack, a common complaint among the officers I see. They get annoyed that I make them go to the hospital every time they call me with these complaints. It is imperative that a therapist knows their limits and makes no assumptions.

It took Bill about three months to come and see me. After all, no one wants to see some "stupid shrink" because "they can't tell me anything that I don't already know." These are the normal statements an officer makes to justify avoiding treatment. The worst issues are the fears of being de-gunned, being labeled as weak or crazy, and fearing that "everyone" will know that they are in therapy. Officers with PTSD are hypervigilant anyway, so none of this other stuff helps make them feel safe to talk.

Hypervigilance is a paranoia based in reality and not fantasy. It comes from the breakdown of healthy defense mechanisms that allow most people to function. Bill had little denial left. His world was not safe. He was hiding behind his drapes in the house and would not let his wife or children out without him. Getting him into my office was difficult. He wanted to know if I thought he was paranoid. I informed him that I believed that one could not be paranoid if one knows what there is to be afraid of. It was clear that he knew what there was to be afraid of.

A debriefing after a critical incident takes me 2–3 hours, and I do not impose time limits. After two hours with Bill, I felt that there was a lot more than I was seeing. His reaction was severe and his symptomatology went beyond a "normal" reaction to such an event. I did what I always do; I went back to any past trauma both on and off the job.

Slowly things were disclosed – each incident he had experienced in his 18 years and had never talked to anyone about because it was "just part of his job." He spoke about the eight-year-old girl who had been hit by a bus and was lying in the street dying. There was nothing he could do for her, so he lay down next to her and held her hand so that she would not die alone. Then there were all the gun calls, the motor vehicle fatalities, and the death notifications. He reviewed each incident and recalled the sights, sounds, and smells. Then he told me of a fatal motor vehicle accident that had happened eleven years ago. His one-month-old son was in the car his wife was driving. She had hit a pole and was killed instantly, but his son had survived. He saw the vehicle and had to identify his wife, who was under the car. He then continued in the same monotone voice, as if he were in a trance, telling me about his sister who had died at the age of four from leukemia and how he was sent to live with his grandmother because his mother was too distraught to handle the other children. He then looked up after almost an hour of nonstop talking of the traumas he had been through and said, "You don't mean stuff like that, do you?"

I am amazed at what people believe is "normal." I looked at him and said, "Yes, that is what I meant." He did not think that any of it played a roll in what he was going through today. I inquired how he had dealt with these "situations" in the past (after all, they were not traumas in his life, at least not at that point). He said he worked more and more and internalized more and more. He had many psychosomatic complaints. I felt these stemmed from the prior history of trauma. I asked him if he had ever thought of or attempted suicide. He said he had thought of it, but would never do it, especially because of his son. I always ask that question, but the most important question is the follow-up one to that: "What is your at-risk behavior, either now or in the past?" The officers typically look at me as if I have two heads. I talk about their excessive speeds to get to a call or not wearing a bulletproof vest when they had in the past. Many departments do not make it mandatory to wear one. I ask about their drinking habits, their drinking and driving habits, driving off-duty habits, spending habits, the amount of sick time and vacation time they have, and whether their call volume has increased or decreased since the incident. There have been many articles published about suicide-by-cop, where a suspect forces the cop to take his life for him (e.g., shooting at officers when he knows that he is out of rounds and still aiming the gun at the officers).

What is rarely spoken about is suicide-by-suspect, when the officer intentionally puts his life in jeopardy hoping that he will be killed in the line of duty. This is the more taboo subject, yet is very realistic. There is glory when officers are killed in the line of duty, as well as financial benefits. The family is taken care of, their children are taken care of, and their house is paid off. There is also little stigma. When I mentioned this to Bill, I finally got some emotions. He was no longer wearing his vest. After his wife was killed, he would drive on the parkway and go as fast as he could, jam on his brakes, and see how close he could get to the sand barriers without hitting them. He took risk after risk, and no one said anything. He had taken three days off because the department made him, but he spoke to no one. This was the first time he spoke of the incidents. He had been involved in many physical altercations over his career and had filed many workman's compensation claims. The number of physical injuries that an officer files over his career appears to be an indicator of past trauma history. People raised in crisis do not do well unless they are in crisis. If it does not find them, they find it. Bill was no exception to this rule.

The department became the secondary trauma as I have seen many times. His chief was gunning for him, and he filed a grievance over the department's decision to not pay him to come for psychological treatment, although they will pay for time when an officer goes for physical treatment. Bill won the grievance, and I won Bill's trust. Bill's chief hates losing and therefore is not too fond of me. Some two years into treatment, Bill came in looking at peace. I asked him what was going on. He told me he had a dream. He dreamt that there were three coffins. His sister who had died was on the left; his dead wife was in the middle; and his grandmother was on the right. His grandmother wanted him to know that she was looking after everyone; his sister wanted him to know that she was having fun; and his first wife wanted him to know that it was not his time, that she wanted him to have a good life and enjoy what he has, and that she would be there when it was his time to come. He said he was OK, that a huge burden had been lifted. He had felt guilty that he had used the life insurance policy to buy things and had always punished himself by not allowing himself to enjoy anything. He was now able to let go of all of that. Over the next few months he got accepted into law school, began enjoying his house and whole family, and no longer was a "road warrior." His passive suicidal tendencies were no longer being played out.

A couple of years later, I got a call at my house from a person who was hyperventilating; it was Bill. He went home, and while I was speaking to him, he told me he was having chest pains and shortness of breath. I told him to go to the hospital. He had gone on a death notification where the family collapsed and everyone became hysterical. He did fine at the scene but subsequently began thinking about what would have happened if the youths had killed him, and his thoughts went on from there. He had projected this family's reaction to what his second wife's reaction would have been as well as to what his mother's reaction was when his sister died. While he was talking, he dropped the phone, which was picked up by his wife. I told her what was going on; that she should have him checked out by a doctor, and that I would see him later.

When he came into the office, he told me a story that he had not told me previously. He remembered going to a call a few weeks after his wife was killed to deal with a fatal motor vehicle accident in which a young woman was hit and killed. Bill requested to do the notification. The husband was home holding their newborn child because the wife had to get some air; she had been in the house for a few weeks since the baby was born. Officer Bill took the infant out of the father's hands, put it on the ground, and told him what happened. He told the father that he would have to come with him to identify the body and asked if he could get someone to watch the baby. The man broke down, but not Officer Bill. He told me he liked watching and causing people as much pain as he had felt. When he told me this story, after several years together over which we had built up a trust, he looked at me and said, "I feel like bursting into tears right now." Officer Bill was finally feeling, something he had needed to do for a lifetime.

Bill is now more susceptible to emotional pain, but he is also more attached to his second wife and two children than he had ever thought he could be. He only needed to see me for a few sessions and was able to get back to work. It is my feeling that if the initial incident had been an isolated incident or if Officer Bill had been debriefed appropriately in the past, then the incidents for which I saw him would have been less traumatic. I believe his trauma history made him a good cop, but it interfered with his attachment to his immediate family. He was clearly a protector and a victim until now.

CASE STUDY: SALLY

Several months ago a recruit called me about a situation she was involved in. "Sally" was concerned about firearms. The firearms section of the academy is the most stressful because this is where recruits typically fail. She told me that prior to coming on the job her department took her to their range to familiarize her with the weapon. While there, a casing from the gun of the recruit next to her hit her in the side of her face and missed her eye by millimeters. She was taken to the hospital, stitched up, and told that she would most likely need plastic surgery.

She said that she was having problems sleeping and was waking up a lot. I asked her if she was waking up every 3–4 hours, feeling anxious, racing heart, sweating, but unable to remember her dream. She was very surprised that I knew that. I have been doing this for so long that I have found that most people can make it though the first dream cycle but not the second one.

My patients think I am clairvoyant, but this is where "you can't not know what you know" comes into play. I asked Sally if she had told anyone, but she said that her department told her not to. I asked her if the director or the range master was informed of what had happened so that they could deal with issues that might occur during the firearms training and qualifications. She said "no." I told her that it is better to let them know prior to her possible failing. She was wavering. She wanted to be a good girl and listen to her department. I told her to call Workman's Compensation and inform them that she was experiencing psychological issues indicative of the diagnosis PTSD. When she called back, she said that her chief and captain called her in and asked what was going on. They both sugar-coated her symptoms, berated her for not being able to handle what she had been through, and told her that this would not be a good way to begin a career. She informed them that she had spoken to me and that I had told her to open the compensation claim for her psychological injuries. I had done this to ensure her a salary for the next year and hold her position as a regular officer should she fail firearms. It would also protect her should she be exposed to any other trauma involving a weapon down the line. She informed me that she was just "going to see what happens."

Sally did not tell the director or the range master and did not give me permission to contact them. Nothing was done. Before she hung up the phone, I reminded her that the "only person who is going to take care of you is you." She gave me the respectful, "I know." I told her that from what I knew about her I felt she had a prior history of being a victim and had learned to do nothing. I encouraged her that no matter what the outcome, she should deal with this because the pattern would likely repeat itself unless she got help. She started to cry. The next call was her telling me that she had failed firearms and the academy and that she would continue to dispatch for the department. She told me she was sure that things happen for a reason.

Herman (1992) talks about why survivors are often revictimized. Survivors have great difficulty protecting themselves in intimate relationships.

Desperate longing for nurturance and care makes it difficult to establish safe and appropriate boundaries with others. The tendency to denigrate oneself and to idealize those to whom one becomes attached further clouds judgment. Empathic attunement to the wishes of others and unconscious habits of obedience make the victim vulnerable to people in positions of power or authority. The dissociative defensive style makes it difficult for the person to form conscious and accurate assessments of danger. The victim's wish to relive the dangerous situation and make it come out right may lead him or her into re-enactments of the abuse (Herman, 1992).

I am unsure if Sally would have made a good police officer. A person who cannot pull a trigger or who hesitates in doing so should not be in law enforcement. I have been exposed to far too many tales of officers left to die because their fellow officers could not use deadly force. These are the ones who are lucky enough to be alive to tell the story.

CASE INVOLVING THREE OFFICERS

One of the most interesting cases I have been involved with ultimately brought three officers into my office. This incident changed many lives, not because of the incident itself, but because of what was uncovered about the officers' lives. I received a call from a distressed police officer. The officer reported difficulty sleeping and numbness. He was avoiding talking about the situation and was very angry about not being taken off of the case when he asked to be.

Case Study: Bob

When this officer, "Bob," came into my office, he said he was working on a case that involved a sergeant from his department. The sergeant and his wife were accused of sexually deviant behavior with minors. Bob was approached by a student who disclosed that the sergeant's wife had molested her while the sergeant watched. He took this information to his superior, who then briefed the Prosecutor's Office, and they made it clear that he was to remain on the case. He tried to speak with the investigator to have him removed because of the intimacy of the case, but he was refused. He was present at the scene after the sergeant and his wife killed themselves. He has vivid memories of the death scene.

Someone had tipped off the sergeant, and he went home where he and his wife took their lives.

Bob has a lot of issues surrounding this outcome. He has issues of feeling responsible as well as questioning his judgment. He has survived on being a good judge of character, and this comes into play when he did not see the behavior of one of their own. He was very distraught to learn all the circumstances surrounding their death. They also left a three-year-old child behind. There is no greater stressor than when another officer takes his or her own life, particularly if you feel you were partially responsible for it. It was also disturbing to learn that the couple had been into sexually deviant behavior and that the potential victims and their abusers remained in the community. He had been using alcohol to numb his pain and memories and was exhibiting signs of at-risk behavior. Officer Bob still has contact with the girl who did the consensual intercept. As the case progressed, Bob's background was delved into, and it was learned that his father had died several years back and that they had had a very tumultuous relationship which included a history of physical and verbal abuse. His mother has remarried and is in a loving relationship, and he refers to his stepfather as "Dad." He was in a relationship with a drug-addicted wife and prior to that had been married as well. He seemed to get into situations that were compromising both on and off the job. He was a heavy drinker who had gotten himself into trouble and given himself a reckless and crazy reputation.

This incident was his 20th mile in a marathon, when no matter how much you have eaten, and how well you have trained, you hit the "wall." Bob was weepy, had concentration and memory difficulties, and was unable to sleep more than a few hours a night. He disclosed having been in therapy before and having ended up in sexual relationship with his therapist. We discussed the timing of the affair and that his ex-wife who was also in a session with the therapist found out about the affair some time afterward and was talking about filing a board complaint. Although we discussed this, it was too soon to deal with this issue. He was going to file a workman's compensation claim with his employer because of the incident. He was concerned about the repercussions.

After much discussion, he filed the claim. SCIBAL, his workman's compensation carrier, and his specific joint insurance fund (JIF) are overseen by a specific individual who was known to deny any and all psychological claims. This was no exception. Discussions with the vice president of SCIBAL clarified why claims for PTSD were having such a difficult time getting approved without having to go to court. This gentleman is a Vietnam veteran who saw combat. As he told me, he did not need to go to ground zero; he sees it every day when he gets up. He thinks that "they knew what they were getting into when they took the job." This is a common response from veterans.

Police officers with prior military experience seem to do better on the job. The population that should have the highest suicide rate among the rank and file does not. Officers between the ages of 55 and 65 are not among those that are killing themselves; it is the younger officers with less than 10 years on the job (Violanti, 2003).

Military personnel are trained differently than police officers. They are trained to kill the enemy, whereas officers are trained to stop the threat. Military personnel normally do not see the faces of the people they kill, whereas police officers are involved in shootings that usually happen at close range. The need to return soldiers to the field as soon as possible has also been recognized (Grinker & Spiegel, 1945). Soldiers do not go home to sleep at night with their families; their families are their comrades in their platoon.

Police officers are not at war, nor do they take a police job to go to war. They take the job because they think they can help someone as well as for the excitement. They expect to go home every night. They do not have a military mentality. This must be understood by those judging them by military standards. Bob and I discussed his needs and how this incident affected his life. We decided to contact the business administrator (BA) because his chief was a known dinosaur that did not believe in psychological services. I spoke with the BA several times, and he proved to be ineffective in taking care of Bob. Contact with the chief reinforced everything I was told he would be and more. He carried on about how officers are today and how they need to grow up and stop complaining. He wanted to know why Bob was having such a difficult time with everything. I explained it to him. He then said, "You should only know what I've been through, and then you'd know trauma." His behavior made me believe that I did know what he had been through. With nothing to lose, I described to him how his behavior was indicative of that associated with being sexually abused. There was silence. He changed his tone and said he had never told anyone. I told him to read the Fraternal Order of Police newspaper that month because the Dear Steph column I write addressed that issue. I encouraged him to see me and to file a workman's compensation claim. He was numb to everything. The incident had not affected him at all, which is why he knew he was in trouble. He did tell me he had noticed a lot of significant positive changes in Bob and so had his coworkers. He said he would do everything in his power to have Bob's claim covered and would think about coming up to see me as well. He told me I could tell Bob we spoke, but that his issues would remain confidential. I had assured him of this.

When I met with Bob, I told him the conversation had gone well and that the chief was very supportive of treatment. The chief had also made it clear that Bob was to use a township vehicle when he came to see me on township time because the incident had happened on duty. He would do all he could to have the claim validated. Bob was thrilled. As time passed, Bob became less symptomatic of PTSD and was able to function better than he had in a long time. He was now dealing with his at-risk behavior, and, after a few months, I found out he had a sense of humor, which had been a casualty of the incident. He had been considering leaving the force, but he was a superb officer.

Bob was frustrated at having been passed over twice for promotions as well as having gotten booted from the detective bureau by a corrupt sergeant. The sergeant is currently under investigation, and Bob has been somewhat vindicated. Bob is no longer a victim. He has taken his third Sergeant examination and awaits the results. He is well respected in the department and has learned to use all the communication tools that have been given to him. He is communicating appropriately and has learned that confrontation is not a bad word; it is a tool to set boundaries and communicate appropriately without having a "temper tantrum." He has been able to get his life back into order and has put the case into its proper perspective. There are still triggers that bring him back to the incident, but through therapy he has learned to deal with them. As with many officers that are involved in critical incidents, once they have dealt with the symptoms, they choose to stay on the force to better themselves. Officer Kevin King, who was on *A&E Investigative Reports* with me when they did the series on "Cop Counselors" in July 2001, says at the end of the show, "I go into your home and help you; why can't I do the same for me?"

Case Study: Mary

Several months later, "Mary," the officer who had been in charge of the investigation and the consensual intercept, came to see me. She also reported sleep, concentration, and memory difficulties. She was crying and found herself falling apart, which she had not done before. She described herself as a "rock," and that she was. She did not understand why this incident had unraveled her as it had. What she was going to get in therapy was far more than she bargained for. I had spoken to Mary on the phone just after the incident. It took her about 2 months to come and see me because of the red tape. She appeared very professional and unsure of what to expect. I had been seeing a friend of hers, so it was easier to establish trust. She told me that she had been heading up sex crimes most of her career. I asked her "Why sex crimes?" She said that most female law enforcement officers are put in sex crimes or the juvenile detective bureau. After several repetitions, she asked, "Do you want me to tell you I was molested?" I told her the reason for my question and the profile of an officer. She began to cry and told me that she had been molested and had not told anyone before.

As the sessions progressed, Mary and I explored all her cases. What was so unnerving to her was that one of her own had done this. She had refused to let Bob off of the case. She had a hard time believing that wolves wear sheep's clothes and needed to accept that sometimes good cops do bad things. Over time, she developed a voice at work and sought legal counsel in case her office attempted to pass her over. She was promoted to lieutenant while working with me.

Mary was able to open up and talk about her abuse although she could not remember who her perpetrator was. She knew that there had been several instances of abuse over time as well as a rape in high school. I told her that in time, when she was ready, it would come to her, most likely in a dream. One week she told me I was right. She told me she had a dream and was able to see the perpetrator, and that she was much younger than she had thought. She was able to tell her children what happened to her and why she raised them the way she did. She has let herself be more vulnerable to those she is close to. She has gained control of a life she had never had in the past. She made a decision to be an educator, which is one of the most difficult things she has done to date.

In September of 2002, Mary taught with me at the police academy. She talked about the case and explained what had come out of it for her. She spoke of her abuse and how it had affected her life, and she did not even know it. After all, she was a rock, and "a rock feels no pain." She was emotional when she was speaking. Her history had allowed her to detach for so many years on the job that no matter what she saw it did not affect her. The understanding that the person one should have been able to trust the most had betrayed her at a very early age triggered an unconscious response from which she could not run. She told the recruits that she felt that she could have been debriefed by someone else and would have been done with it in a month or so, but she told them she did not think there was another person she could have seen in the world that would have addressed her abuse history and made sense of her reaction. She told me that opening up and communicating led to her daughter asking her to be in the delivery room with her when she delivered her baby. While her daughter was giving birth, she was in a lot of pain and turned to Mary for guidance. Mary said, "The old me would have told her to 'suck it up and bare it, we have all had to go through this,'" but instead she was able to say, "Honey, just concentrate on that beautiful baby and the gift you get to take home; we'll get through this together." With tears in my eyes, I knew I had done my job.

Mary's prior trauma had helped her on the job. She had been able to go to any crime scene, no matter how gruesome or traumatic, and detach and do a thorough investigation. On the way home she would not think twice about what she had just seen. Today, she will do the same thorough job, detach while at the scene, and then feel afterwards in a safe and appropriate place. She is no longer burdened with keeping the feelings inside.

Case Study: Chief Fuzzy

The third and most difficult subject in this case was "Fuzzy." His nickname is short for Warm and Fuzzy. He has no consistent emotions. After speaking with him, I received a document in five sections that was 20 pages long. The binder smelled of smoke, which reflected the 3–5 packs of cigarettes he smoked a day. The last page reads,

> Stephanie, I have just read all that I wrote yesterday. All that ran thru my mind all last night. While I still wonder as to why I have exposed so much of myself I fully realize that my finally telling someone who might care simply makes me feel better about it. Not a lot but some. The frustration, the secrecy, the hell, of all of this is unending I realize that holding this inside of me has probably helped in making me so hard, so cold, when it comes to handling those incidents that cause others to become emotional. You're aware of the

Sergeant I had who committed suicide along with his wife. My true reaction? Handle it, it's just another incident. At the scene I had no feelings. I simply did not have any emotions. Wading thru the blood, etc., in the bathroom with two of them lying there simply had no effect on me at all. It was just another suicide. I spent some time trying to determine how the guns were fired and how her front teeth had been blown out of her mouth and onto the floor. She was on her back, face and head blown apart, looking at me. It didn't mean a thing. He was crumpled into the wall with a hole thru his head. And he and I were friends. I was not happy with the time delay between the telephone intercept and when the take down was to occur. I felt very strongly that the possibility of suicide was very, very possible. I could have interceded. I didn't. But knowing that I could have prevented the entire incident has no effect on me. There's no emotion.

This was a direct result of years of abuse and trauma.

Fuzzy started getting physically abused at age 5 by his mom, followed by his brother. This did not happen more than a couple of times. About a year later his sexual abuse or use, as he would say, started with the retarded 35-year-old man who cleaned their house for a dollar. The man could not talk but seemed to be a protector from his brother and his brother's friends. This went on until Fuzzy was about 12 years old. He writes,

> Sometimes I feel like crawling into a corner and just crying. Of course that's neither practical nor beneficial. As a Chief of Police with 31 years of service, can you imagine the utter catastrophe that would occur if anyone, anywhere, knew of my past and my innermost doubts and questions?

I sent him a book called *Knight in Rusty Armor* by R. Fischer (1987) that I make all the recruits read. It seemed to have a profound impact on him. There is a character in the book called Merlin who was the knight's guide. Fuzzy's writings reflected my role in his life when he referred to me as Merlin. It was better than "fuzzy." He writes that he has started to change after reading the book and does not know why. He writes,

> I must conclude that the knowledge that my Merlin has given me provides me with some type of inner confidence. A feeling that maybe, just maybe, I can strip myself of all the hurts, the confusion, the fake personalities, the derived opinions and long-held concepts that have haunted me all of my life. It's as if I had fallen overboard and was just about to accept the fact that I was going to die. Then a single life preserver appeared. Having reached out and grabbed that life preserver, I've greatly increased the chances of survival. Yet the sharks are just below circling. Accept the reality, Merlin. You're that life preserver whether you like it or

not. Considering your personality, one would assume that you (like me) prefer the challenge. Prefer to be the participant rather than the spectator. Prefer to handle that which others would avoid. Prefer to accept the responsibility of the outcome knowing damn full well that no one else would even play the game. Most probably unknown to you is just how close to drowning this individual is/was. Far closer then has been remotely expressed to you. Admittedly that's still a very strong possibility. When long held negative feelings, concepts, responsibilities, failures, and on and on, take total control of one's emotions they become the uncontrollable. They, not the individual, decide the next course that'll be followed. It matters little how intellectual, how educated, how experienced one is. The only alternative is to terminate all that is continually and increasingly ripping one apart. That is not a socially acceptable alternative, but it's the only one that insures an end to pain, fear, and doubt. This game has been dropped into your ballpark. What no one told you was that it's already in the 9th inning. You're in a tie game. The bases are loaded with 2 outs. And the count on the batter is 3 balls and 1 strike. You threw that first strike already, Merlin. Nice pitch. One can only hope that you've got 2 more in that bag-of-tricks of yours. Don't walk'um and don't let'um get a hit either. What do you throw? The curve, the slider, maybe the split-fingered fastball. Possibly just that straight fastball, right down the middle. But if it's a little high, this batter will drive it right out of the park. The next pitch is up to you. It's hell being a pitcher, but that's what you wanted to be . . . so pitch, Merlin.

Pitch I did and still do. It is one of the most difficult cases I have had. Fuzzy is very busy being a chief of a sizeable department with many commitments. My office is over 100 miles away. He comes up for 3 hours each time, so we can cover a lot of material. His wife will not participate in treatment because, according to him, "Her world revolves around my being a chief and her perspective of all that goes with the title." She does not want to address his history, and it continues to isolate him more and more. He was able to communicate with her for about a month. They had sex for the first time in many years and spent every waking hour together. The equilibrium had been altered, but only briefly. At this point things are back to "normal," which means he lives in his head with the demons, and she continues to put him on a pedestal not knowing what is going on in his world.

It is clear that because of his drive to succeed and his not caring about what would happen to him (his fear of death having been removed years ago), he learned to take no prisoners. He was a Navy man who had seen his fair share of critical incidents prior to his police job. He was able to feel physical pain but not emotional pain when we began this process. As of this writing, he is in little to no physical pain, but he now experiences emotional pain, which is harder for him to deal with. He continues to see me and to play ball. Some innings are better than others, but he is a fair player who is willing to share plays. It is evident that his history of trauma and abuse helped him to achieve all that he did on the job, but it adds to his inner turmoil off of the job.

CASE STUDY: STEVE

The last officer I want to profile is a young African-American police officer, "Steve," who sought treatment because of issues with his sexuality. He was acting out with as many as ten different women in a month. He had a steady girlfriend but was unable to commit. It was not uncommon for him to be carrying on two very intense relationships at the same time. Mainly his maternal grandparents, whom he adored, brought him up. The only real emotion shown was for his grandmother. Steve had little contact with his biological father after his early teens. When is father would tell him that he was coming for him, Steve would wait outside, and his father would not show up. The house seemed to be a shelter for the family.

When Steve was 10 years old, he was playing with an older black boy who molested him. There were very few black families in the neighborhood at the time, and this incident would change Steve's outlook on blacks as well. He had been questioning if he was gay, but clearly stated he was not attracted to men. Deep down he felt he should have been able to do something to stop the molestation because he did not believe that he was gay. Within two years, he was molested by his female babysitters dozens of times. As statistics show, this type of abuse is common (Russell, 1984). Steve was not attracted to black women; on a deep level, it had been blacks who had betrayed him the most. First his mother betrayed him by not being able to take care of him emotionally or physically as a child. Then his father betrayed him by abandoning him. And then he was molested by a black male whom he had known. Steve was very abusive to the woman he dated, not physically, but mentally. Steve is one of the most detached men I have in my practice.

It took almost a year of working with him to help him see that what he was doing to the women in his life was similar to what had been done to him as a child. He would "love them and leave them." He was tried on medication for his impulse control issues, but the medicine did not work. He was learning to set boundaries in therapy and had told several family members and friends what had happened to him as a child. He was aware that the person who molested him was dead, so there was no issue of reporting the abuse. Many therapists do not know that there is no statute of limitations for reporting abuse if the person is still alive and may have contact with children.

The more time Steve spent in therapy dealing with his behavior and having consequences associated with the behavior, the less he acted out. He was taking responsibility for his own actions and was having trouble dealing with the pain he had caused so many women. He struggled with how to handle this and was honest with women when they invited him on a date. He was now trying to commit to his long-time girlfriend whom he clearly loved. She was having some medical issues at the time, and the doctors were looking for multiple sclerosis (MS). Steve was aware of the implications if she had the disease. The question that come up in therapy was whether or not he would leave her if she was diagnosed with MS. And, if not, did he want her to think that he asked her because he felt sorry for her? While he was talking to me, he became very emotional. It became clear that he wanted to spend the rest of his life with her. He left my office with ten minutes to spare, went to the jewelry store, and bought her an engagement ring.

Steve was married this past summer and continues to seek psychotherapy and to work on issues of boundary setting as well as thinking of others and not just himself. He is more grounded and has been able to be monogamous since making up his mind to get married. He is better at communicating with others, but he still remains very detached from most emotional situations. This will be a mixed blessing for him should the emotional wall come down. It will be needed, however, to lead an emotionally fulfilled life.

CONCLUSION

In conclusion, officers who come on the job with PTSD do very well. They are the people who seem to get into the most incidents, take the greatest risks on the job, and are more likely to file workman's compensation claims for physical injuries than psychological ones. It is believed that officers who act out through excessive use of force or have more than the average number of citizen complaints against them have a history of abuse and are the abusers. These are the officers that I do not see. The officers I see are the protectors. They are constantly putting themselves in harm's way. They will not steal or lie. They will provoke the perpetrator to hit them first, but they will never strike without cause. They feel very little in the way of emotions and tend to drink more than others. This, I believe, is to drown any feeling that might creep up on them when they least expect it. Nighttime is when the demons come out for them. They have had relationships that are tumultuous and do not know why. They do not realize that they cannot live without chaos. They are the officers this country is proud to call their own. It is time for us to take care of them. An officer who comes on the job with PTSD can be a tremendous asset to a department as long as their etiology has been determined. How people handle stressful situations in childhood is typically how they handle them as an adult. If the child used to be a bully, in all likelihood he will be a bully as an adult. We need to look into these matters to help in the recruitment process of our officers today.

REFERENCES

American Psychiatric Association. (1994). *Diagnostic and Statistical Manual of Mental Disorders* (4th ed.). Washington, DC: APA.

Fisher, R. (1987). *Knight in Rusty Armor.* New York: Wilshire.

Grinker, R. R., & Spiegel, J. (1945). *Men under Stress.* Philadelphia: Blakeston.

Herman, J. L.(1992). *Trauma and Recovery.* New York: Basic Books.

Lenore, T. (1990). *Too Scared to Cry.* New York: Basic Books.

Russell, D. E. H. (1984). *Sexual Exploitation: Rape, Child Sexual Abuse, and Sexual Harassment.* Beverly Hills, CA: Sage.

Violanti, J. M. (2003). *The Buffalo Police Health Pilot Study: Preliminary Results.* Unpublished manuscript.

Chapter 6

TRAUMA TYPE AND FREQUENCY: RISK FACTORS FOR POSTTRAUMATIC STRESS DISORDER IN POLICING

ANNE GEHRKE AND JOHN M. VIOLANTI

INTRODUCTION

Given their frequent assignment to respond to critical and threatening situations, police officers are a high-risk population in terms of exposure to traumatic stress. This risk status is further heightened by their regular exposure to human-initiated violence. Human-initiated traumata cause more severe and more chronic impairment than other types (Maercker, 1997). Most of the critical incidents that police officers deal with are type-I traumata; they are short-term incidents characterized by suddenness, acute life-threat, and surprise. They may also encounter type-II traumata, which are long-term. Both types are considered in this study. Given that trauma in the police occupation is rarely avoidable, it is necessary to focus on prevention to manage traumatic stress risk.

Occupational safety is more than prevention of physical injuries or accidents. It is also concerned with facilitating officers' health, well-being, and professional functioning. The inevitability of officers' confrontation with trauma makes primary prevention difficult but highlights the need for secondary prevention. To implement secondary prevention strategies, one has to know the specific traumatic stress risk factors. This chapter describes an empirical analysis of specific risk factors, as well as protective factors, in the police occupation. The models developed may be useful for preventive and supportive interventions in training recruits, psychological assessment, psychological precautions, and follow-up care of police officers.

Despite the incidence of exposure to extreme situations and traumatic experiences, the fact that only a small proportion of officers develop posttraumatic stress disorder (PTSD) is testament to their stress resilience (Lucas, 2000). It also indicates a need to understand the protective factors that facilitate such outcomes. This prompts the question: Which factors help an employee to stay healthy and to cope successfully with traumatic experiences? Once identified, this knowledge could be used to develop effective intervention strategies. This chapter examines the influence of (1) the type and (2) the frequency of a traumatic incident on traumatic stress risk. However, a key focus here is on how potentially protective factors may mediate this relationship.

Pieper & Maercker (1999) note that mortality and suicide risk were higher among trauma victims who did not seek professional help. The suicidal act reflects extreme helplessness and is a result of a deficit of adaptive coping mechanisms. Strong police cultural values (i.e. masculinity and patriarchal attitudes, control of affective responses to distressing circumstances, effectiveness and competitiveness, helper stereotype and authority) intensify these aspects and the self-destructive behavior. Increased alcohol use and abuse is an additional significant problem within this occupation. The ritual of social drinking after work provides positive reinforcement for the tendency to solve problems by alcohol and to use alcohol to relax. Alcohol abuse and its symptoms may lead to inability to work. Pieper & Maercker (1999) also mention a higher rate of early retirements. The wish to retire may be an extreme solution and may be seen as an "all or nothing" decision.

A demographic risk factor is gender (Davis & Breslau, 1998; Halligan & Yehuda, 2000; Kessler, Sonnega, Bromet, Hughes, & Nelson, 1995; Maercker, 1997). The prevalence of PTSD is typically higher in women than in men. Protective and supportive factors must also be considered.

Hardiness (Kobasa, 1979) has regularly been implicated in this context. Hardy persons tend to have dedication to a purpose, a sense of control over situations, and a perception of events as challenges rather than threats. Allen (1995) states that "the availability of social support and the capacity to make use of it can protect traumatized persons from developing PTSD" (p. 186). This statement emphasizes both the need for social support to be available within and outside the organization and the need for officers to be able to make use of it as they interact in a social network. In the present study, perceived and received social support, as well as social interaction, are examined with regard to their protective influence on traumatic stress risk.

Evidence for an influence of age on traumatic stress risk has been inconsistent. Some studies show that being younger at the time of trauma increases PTSD risk (Green, 1994). However, in a meta-analytic study, Brewin, Andrews, and Valentine (2000) conclude that age does not influence the risk of PTSD and suggest that earlier support for this relationship may have been due to a confoundation of design and outcomes. Brown, Fielding, and Grover (1999) conclude that living single or with a partner has no significant influence for the stress risk in either women or men (measured by the General Health Questionnaire). However, Halligan and Yehuda (2000) conclude that being divorced or widowed is a risk factor. The variable "marital status" is included as a protective influence on traumatic stress risk, as are the variables "hardiness," "perceived and actual social support," and "social interaction." In regard to vulnerabilities, Lucas' (2000) finding of a relationship between cumulating stressful events and psychological difficulties leads to "job activity level" and "life events added in the past year" being examined as factors. Variables such as age, marital status, years served as a police officer, job activity level, social interactions, perceived and actual received social support, the life events added in the past year, as well hardiness, play a mediating role.

VARIABLES

Dependent Variable – Criterion

The dependent variable was traumatic stress, with the dimensions high versus low. A binary version of the total score from the "Impact of Event Scale" (Horowitz, Wilner, & Alvarez, 1979) was calculated to use it as dependent variable.

Independent Variables

Three independent variables were included: trauma type, its frequency, and the participant's gender. The variable trauma type was divided into 9 subcategories: a shooting involving a colleague (PIS1), involvement in a shooting oneself (PIS2), and seeing abused children (PIS3), victims of serious traffic accidents (PIS4), someone die (PIS5), dead bodies (PIS6), severely assaulted victims (PIS7), or homicide victims (PIS8). The last category was named "other disturbing incidents" (PIS9). Various situations were included or rather have been described by police officers as "other disturbing incidents." They mentioned animal abuse, suicides, rape victims, elderly abuse, domestic violence, and narcotics addiction. The variable "trauma type" was registered by the question if the officer experienced the incident in the past year or not. The frequencies of each of these incident types over the past year were recorded. The frequencies were used as a second group of independent variables. Table 6-1 shows the frequencies of trauma types experienced in the present sample.

Mediating Variables

The mediating role of several variables was examined. These were age, marital status, years served as a police officer, police work activity level, perceived and instrumental social support, social interactions, and life events added in the past year. "Police work activity level" was represented by the three categories: low, moderate, and high workload. "Perceived social support" referred to the degree to which the person perceives that he/she has social support, whereas "Instrumental social support" referred to actual social support received (i.e., support that has been given in some way). "Social interaction" was scored in terms of the number of people within the social network with whom the police officer regularly was in contact, visited, and socialized. "Life events added in the past year" included all critical incidents except the traumatic ones (e.g., marriage or divorce, children being born, or moving out). The moderating variable "hardiness" was measured with the "Hardiness Scale, Short Version" (Bartone, 1995).

SAMPLE

The random sample consisted of 115 police officers from the Buffalo, New York Police Department. Sample demographics are recorded in Table 6-2.

TABLE 6-1
FREQUENCIES OF TRAUMA TYPES

	Females (N = 45)		Males (N = 70)		Entire Sample (N = 115)	
Incident Type Experienced	*Yes*	*No*	*Yes*	*No*	*Yes*	*No*
(PIS1) Shooting involving a colleague	8 (17.8%)	37 (82.2%)	16 (22.9%)	54 (77.1%)	24 (20.9%)	91 (79.1%)
(PIS2) Involvement in a shooting oneself	4 (8.9%)	41 (91.1%)	13 (18.6%)	57 (81.4%)	17 (14.8%)	98 (85.2%)
(PIS3) Seeing abused children	27 (60.0%)	18 (40.0%)	51 (72.9%)	19 (27.1%)	78 (67.8%)	37 (32.2%)
(PIS4) Victims of serious traffic accident	17 (37.8%)	28 (62.2%)	36 (51.4%)	34 (48.6%)	53 (46.1%)	62 (53.9%)
(PIS5) Seeing someone die	12 (26.7%)	33 (73.3%)	27 (38.6%)	43 (61.4%)	39 (33.9%)	76 (66.1%)
(PIS6) Victims of serious traffic accident	27 (60.0%)	18 (40.0%)	44 (62.6%)	26 (37.1%)	71 (61.7%)	44 (38.3%)
(PIS7) Severely assaulted victims	25 (55.6%)	20 (44.4%)	51 (72.9%)	19 (27.1%)	76 (66.1%)	39 (33.9%)
(PIS8) Victims of homicide	17 (37.8%)	28 (62.2%)	37 (52.9%)	33 (47.1%)	54 (47.0%)	61 (53.0%)
(PIS9) Other disturbing incidents	16 (35.6%)	29 (64.4%)	36 (51.4%)	34 (48.6%)	52 (45.2%)	63 (54.8%)

TABLE 6-2
CHARACTERISTICS OF POLICE SAMPLE

		Females (N = 45)	Males (N = 70)
Age (Mean)		38.96 (SD 6.30)	39.94 (SD 8.24)
Race (in %)	Caucasian	75.4	70.0
	African	24.4	18.6
	Hispanic	–	11.4
Marital status (in %)	Never married	26.7	17.1
	Married	48.9	68.6
	Divorced/separated	22.2	8.6
	Divorced remarried	–	4.3
	Living with someone	2.2	1.4
Years served as police officer (Mean)		10.7 (SD 6.52)	15.14 (SD 9.53)
Police work activity level (in %)	High work load	46.7	62.9
	Moderate work load	33.3	35.7
	Low work load	20.0	1.4

PROCEDURE

Data was collected at the Center for Preventive Medicine, State University of New York at Buffalo, School of Medicine and Biomedical Science. A total of 115 sworn police officers were randomly selected using a computer-generated random number table. All officers had an equal probability of being selected, including those on vacation; personnel on personal leave or sick leave were included in the sample selection. Sampling was stratified by race and gender to ensure a representative sample. Selected officers were contacted for a brief interview to explain the study, procedures, benefits, and risks involved. Participants were required to sign an informed consent form if they agreed to take part. Officers who declined were replaced by a second sampling. This process was continued until the desired number of participants was obtained. The sampling procedure resulted in a 100% response rate.

Measures

The Impact of Event Scale (IES) (Horowitz et al., 1979) was used to assess the psychological effect of trauma exposure. Sundin and Horowitz (2002) argue caution in its use because, although it includes the dimensions avoidance and intrusion, it does not include the symptom cluster "hyperarousal" contained in the PTSD diagnosis in DSM-IV. Notwithstanding, they emphasize that the IES remains a useful measure of stress reactions after a range of traumatic events. According to Sundin and Horowitz (2002), the internal consistency of intrusion has a mean of $\alpha = 0.86$ and of avoidance a mean $\alpha = 0.82$. The subscales represent homogeneous constructs that discriminate between severe and mild stress reactions (Sundin & Horowitz, 2002).

"Hardiness" was measured with the "Hardiness Scale, Short Version" (Bartone, 1995). This short, 15-item version includes items covering the three dimensions of commitment, control, and challenge. It has good psychometric properties and has demonstrated validity with several samples including soldiers exposed to combat stressors.

"Trauma type" was measured by questioning. The variable was registered using the categories "experienced yes" or "no." In addition, the participants described their experiences. The descriptions were collected separately in category PIS10 (string variable). The frequencies of each incident type over the past year were counted by (and for) every participant.

"Perceived social support" refers to the degree to which the person perceives that he/she has social support. It was measured by a 3-point scale "0" for "never," "1" for "sometimes," and "2" for "always." The higher the score, the more support was perceived. "Instrumental social support" refers to actual social support received. It means that support has been given in some way. It was measured "yes" or "no." The score was the number of "yes" answers, meaning that they did receive some kind of actual support from others. The "demographic variables" age, gender, marital status, years served as police officer, and police work activity level were registered by questionnaires or structured interviews.

Statistical Analyses

To demonstrate if incident type and frequency as well as moderator variables can be used to predict a PTSD risk in police officers, several logistic regression models were calculated. The logistic regressions were performed backwards stepwise with the Likelihood Ratio-method because stepwise regression is usually performed in the exploratory phase of research or for purposes of pure prediction.

In consideration of the sample size, the missing values were calculated by the means of the sample to maintain the entire sample.

The variable "IES total score" (IEPTSD) was recoded into a binary variable to use it as dependent variable. The two categories of the dependent variable "IES total dichotomy" (IESRISK) were specified as "low risk" and "high risk" by calculating the mean of the IES total score. The label "low" has a value of 1 and reflects the data below the mean. Label "high" has a value of 2 and stands for the scores above the mean.

Some moderator variables (e.g., age, years served as police officer) were transformed into categorical data to reduce the variety of information. Individual diversity would have been wider using the original data. Nevertheless, in consideration of the sample size and the quantity of variables, the scope of data would have been too extensive.

The frequencies for each variable and its dimensions were calculated. Categories were formed by using percentiles (25%, 50%, 75%). The number of officers in each category was equal; thus altering the boundaries was necessary in some cases. Eventually variables were recoded into new ones with the calculated categories.

"Age" was converted into the four categories: ≤ 33 years old (1), ≤ 39 years old (2), ≤ 45 years old (3), and > 45 years (4). The variable "years served" was divided into the following four categories: ≤ 6 years (1), ≤ 13 years (2), ≤ 17 years (3), and > 17 years (4). For "social interactions" (defined by the number of persons interacted with on a regular basis within the respondents' social environment), four categories were specified: ≤ 10 (1), ≤ 16 (2), ≤ 26 (3), and > 26 (4). Three categories were calculated for the variable "life events" (defined as the number of negative life events experienced by the respondent within the past year): no significant life events (1), 1–2 life events (2), and ≥ 3 life events (3). "Perceived social support" (actions of others perceived as supportive by the respondent) was reflected by two categories: "low" (scores from 14 to 20) and high (score 21). "Instrumental support" (actions actually performed by others that the respondent considered to be supportive) was divided into two categories as well. "Low" reflects scores 5–11, and "high" stands for scores from 12–19.

RESULTS

Prevalence

Lifetime prevalence for developing a posttraumatic stress disorder (PTSD) in the general population is declared to be 1 to 14% (American Psychiatric Association, 1999). In the present sample of 115 police officers, the prevalence for high risk of PTSD was found to be higher than in the general population. According to DSM-IV (American Psychiatric Association, 1999) studies on risk populations (e.g., veterans, victims of criminal violence) resulted in a prevalence of 3 to 58%.

Cross tables of "IES risk" and "life events added over the past year" were calculated to illustrate risks and prevalence (table 6-3). Forty-nine of 115 persons were under high traumatic stress risk, which is a prevalence of 42.5% for this sample. Only four persons, who did not experience any critical life events, recorded high stress risk. Thus, the risk of having a high IES score was 30.8% for police officers who have not been exposed to any life events in the past. Officers who experienced 1 or 2 life events had a risk of 32.7%, and participants with 3 or more life events in the past year had a risk of 56%. Calculation of relative stress risk revealed that persons exposed to critical life events before had a 1.4 times higher risk than participants without any life events in the past year.

TABLE 6-3
CROSS TABLES OF "IMPACT OF EVENT SCALE RISK" AND
"LIFE EVENTS ADDED OVER THE PAST YEAR"

			Categories of Life Events			Total
			No Life Event (1)	1–2 Life Events (2)	3 Life Events (3)	
IES	Low risk (1)	Number	9	35	22	66
dichotomy		% of category	69.2%	67.3%	44.0%	57.4%
	High risk (2)	Number	4	17	28	49
		% of category	30.8%	32.7%	56.0%	42.6%
Total		Number	13	52	50	115
		% of category	100.0%	100.0%	100.0%	100.0%

Trauma Type

Regression analysis included the following independent variables: a shooting in which a colleague was involved, involvement in a shooting oneself, seeing abused children, victims of serious traffic accidents, someone die, dead bodies, severely assaulted victims, and homicide victims, as well as "other disturbing incidents." Gender was used as an independent variable in the present study to distinguish between the impact of trauma on female and male officers. Therefore, regression models for trauma types were performed for female and male participants separately.

Entire Sample

The final model "trauma type" shows that only one category of the examined traumatic events has a significant influence on the risk of developing a PTSD in the entire sample. The events, which have been included in "other disturbing incidents," increased the risk of PTSD significantly (p = 0.031) by a factor of 2.440 (confidence interval 1.086 to 5.483). Three other dimensions of traumatic incidents were included in the final model even though their influence was not statistically significant.

Officers who dealt with abused children recorded a 2.393 times higher traumatic stress risk (confidence interval 0.950 to 6.032, p = 0.064) compared with officers who had not. Participants who reported seeing someone die were 1.508 times more likely to record high stress scores than officers who did not (confidence interval 0.551 to 4.126, p = 0.424). Being confronted with homicide victims increased traumatic stress risk by a factor of 1.744 (confidence interval 0.666 to 4.564, p = 0.257).

No influence was evident for the following traumatic events: shooting involving a colleague, involvement in a shooting oneself, seeing victims of serious traffic accidents, seeing dead bodies, and seeing severely assaulted victims. Thus, these incident types were excluded from the final model for the influence of the type of traumatic incident on traumatic stress risk. The final model predicts traumatic stress risk correctly for 67% of all cases. High risk is predicted correctly in 67.3% of all participants.

Female Participants

The final regression model "trauma type" for female participants differs from the final model for the entire sample. Five regression coefficients form this final model; three were statistically significant. The included incident types are witnessing a shooting involving a colleague, seeing abused children, seeing someone die, being confronted with severely assaulted victims, and other disturbing incidents. The category "other disturbing incidents" had the greatest influence on this final regression model. The odds ratio is 35.056 (confidence interval 2.932 to 420.431, p = 0.005). Therefore, traumatic incidents within this category increase the traumatic stress risk by a factor of 35 in female officers. The odds ratio for an officer who experienced a shooting involving a colleague is 0.038 (confidence interval 0.002 to 0.710, p = 0.029). Thus this incident type decreases the risk for women in this sample. A significant influence on stress risk was evident for "seeing abused children." Female participants who experienced confrontations with abused children within the past year are under a 32.913 higher risk (confidence interval 2.175 to 498.038, p = 0.012) than officers who did not. The traumatic incident of seeing someone die increases the risk of PTSD for a female officer by a factor of 4.238 (confidence interval 0.674 to 26.632, p = 0.124). An odds ratio of 0.079 (confidence interval 0.004 to 1.411, p = 0.084) was evident for the incident type "severely assaulted victims," which decreases the risk for development of PTSD in female officers. No influence was found for the following: involved in a shooting oneself, victims of serious traffic accidents, dead bodies, as well as confrontation with victims of homicide. Consequently, these trauma types were excluded from the final model. The final model predicts the risk of PTSD correctly for 80% of all cases. High risk is predicted correctly in 77.8% cases of all participants.

Male Participants

The final model "trauma type" for male participants revealed that two out of nine traumatic incidents had a significant influence on traumatic stress risk. The trauma type "colleague involved in a shooting" puts male officers under a 4.422 times higher risk, compared with an officer who did not experience such a trauma over the past year (confidence interval 1.148 to 17.028, p = 0.031). Confrontation with "victims of homicide" increased risk significantly (p = 0.019) by a factor of 15.560 (confidence interval 1.566 to 154.630). In addition, the final model includes two other types, even though their influence was not statistically significant.

Officers who dealt with "abused children" recorded a 3.069 times higher traumatic stress risk (confidence interval 0.885 to 10.650, p = 0.77) compared with officers who did not. An odds ratio of 0.131 (confidence interval 0.013 to 1.351, p = 0.088) was evident for the trauma type "dead bodies," which therefore decreases stress risk in male officers.

No influence was found for the following traumatic events: being involved in a shooting oneself, seeing victims of serious traffic accidents, seeing someone die, seeing severely assaulted victims, as well as other disturbing incidents. Thus, these incident types were excluded from the final model for the influence of the type of traumatic incident on traumatic stress risk. The final model predicts the risk of PTSD correctly for 70% of all cases. High risk is predicted correctly in 67.7% of all participants. The models are summarized in Table 6-4.

Trauma Type and Frequency

The independent variables used to calculate a model for the influence of incident type and the frequency of a traumatic event on traumatic stress risk were the incident types listed above, as well as their frequencies over the past year. Calculations were performed only for the entire sample and for male participants; the number of female participants was too small for the quantity of variables to calculate logistic regression.

Entire Sample

The final model "incident type and frequency" revealed an influence of the following variables: colleague involved in a shooting, seeing abused children, other disturbing incidents, frequency of shootings involving a colleague over the past year, frequency of seeing abused children over the past year, frequency over the past year of seeing someone die, frequency over the past year of being confronted with severely assaulted victims, as well as frequency of seeing homicide victims over the past year. Only "other disturbing incidents" and "frequency of shootings in which a colleague was involved over the past year" were statistically significant.

The traumatic event "colleague involved in a shooting" decreased stress risk by a factor of 0.466 (confidence interval 0.108 to 2.021, p = 0.308). Confrontation with abused children over the past year increased

TABLE 6-4
ODDS RATIOS FOR HIGH RISK OF POSTTRAUMATIC STRESS DISORDER
MEASURED BY THE IMPACT OF EVENT SCALE (HOROWITZ ET AL., 1979) –
FINAL MODELS "TRAUMA TYPE"

	Model: Females (N = 45)			Model: Males (N = 70)			Model: Entire Sample (N = 115)		
Incident Type	Exp(B)	Confidence		Exp(B)	Confidence		Exp(B)	Confidence	
(PIS1) Colleague involved in shooting	0.038*	0.002	0.710	4.42*	1.14	17.02			
(PIS2) Involved in shooting oneself									
(PIS3) Seeing abused children	32.91*	2.175	498.03	3.06	0.885	10.65	2.39	0.950	6.02
(PIS4) Victims of serious traffic accident									
(PIS5) Seeing someone die	4.23	0.674	26.63				1.50	0.551	4.12
(PIS6) Dead bodies				0.13	0.013	1.351			
(PIS7) Severely assaulted victims	0.07	0.004	1.411						
(PIS8) Victims of homicide				15.56*	1.56	154.6	1.74	0.666	4.56
(PIS9) Other disturbing incidents	35.05**	2.923	420.43				2.44*	1.08	5.48
–2LL	39.103			79.403			138.667		
Change in –2LL	21.468**			16.721**			18.235**		
Class table % OK	80.0			70.0			67.0		
% Predicted high risk	77.8			67.7			67.3		
Goodness of FIT	Chi – Square 5.918			Chi – Square 4.531			Chi – Square 6.437		
(Hosmer-Lemeshow)	Significance 0.314			Significance 0.605			Significance 0.376		

Significance: * p < 0.05; ** p < 0.01; ***p < 0.001

traumatic stress risk by 2.456 times compared with participants not so exposed (confidence interval 0.771 to 7.824, p = 0.129). For the category "other disturbing incidents" an odds ratio of 3.495 (confidence interval 1.413 to 8.644, p = 0.007) was calculated within this model.

The frequency of shootings involving a colleague increased traumatic stress risk by a factor of 2.650 (confidence interval 1.015 to 6.918, $p = 0.047$). Thus, every time an officer experiences a shooting involving a colleague, his stress risk increases by a factor of 2.650 relative to officers who were not confronted with this type of event. A 1.041 (confidence interval 0.967 to 1.120, $p = 0.288$) times higher risk of developing a PTSD was shown in terms of the frequency of seeing abused children over the past year, which is an odds ratio of nearly 1 and therefore of limited significance. A 1.257 times higher risk was calculated for the frequency of seeing someone die (confidence interval 0.884 to 1.786, $p = 0.202$). The odds ratio for the trauma frequency of being confronted with severely assaulted victims over the past year was 0.991 (confidence interval 0.956 to 1.027, $p = 0.605$), which is almost 1 and therefore no has meaningful influence on the risk of developing a PTSD. The frequency of experiencing a confrontation with victims of homicide increases the risk of PTSD by a factor of 1.189 (confidence interval 0.984 to 1.437, $p = 0.073$). The final model predicts the risk of PTSD correctly for 65.3% of all cases. High risk was predicted correctly in 74.8% of all officers.

Male Participants

The final regression model "trauma type & frequency" for male participants differs from that for the entire sample. The model consists of seven regression coefficients, four of which are statistically significant. The included incident types are: a colleague has been involved in a shooting, victims of a serious traffic accident, dead bodies, other disturbing incidents, frequency of seeing abused children over the past year, frequency over the past year of being confronted with severely assaulted victims, as well as the frequency over the past year of dealing with homicide victims. The following variables were statistically significant within the final model for male participants: colleague involved in a shooting, victims of a serious traffic accident, dead bodies, and frequency over the past year of being confronted with homicide victims.

The category "victims of serious traffic accidents" was highly influential within this final regression model. The odds ratio for this trauma type was 5.350 (confidence interval 1.048 to 27.306, $p = 0.044$). The odds ratio for an officer who experienced a shooting involving his colleague was 4.138 (confidence interval 1.065 to 16.071, p = 0.040). The incident type "dead bodies" decreases the risk for male officers because its odds ratio was 0.118 (confidence interval 0.017 to 0.819, p = 0.031). An influence on traumatic stress risk was also evident for the category "other disturbing incidents." Traumata included in this category increase risk by a factor of 2.930 (confidence interval 0.797 to 10.774, p = 0.106). The frequency of confrontations with abused children within the past year puts male officers under a 1.067 higher risk (confidence interval 0.984 to 1.156, p = 0.114) than officers who did not have this experience, which is almost 1 and therefore a similar result as in the model for the entire sample. An odds ratio of 0.970 (confidence interval 0.924 to 1.018, p = 0.223) was shown for the frequency of incident type "severely assaulted victims" over the past year, which is almost 1 but decreases risk in male officers slightly. The frequency of confrontations with homicide victims over the past year increases risk by a factor of 1.769 (confidence interval 1.137 to 2.753, p = 0.011) in male officers. The final model predicts traumatic stress risk correctly for 80% of all cases. High risk is predicted correctly in 74.28% cases of all participants. The models are summarized below in Table 6-5.

Mediating Variables

Due to the sample size and number of variables, logistic regression for hypothesized "mediating variables" only was performed for the entire sample. In addition to the independent variables used in the calculation of the model "incident type and frequency over the past year," the following mediating variables were included: age, gender, marital status, years of service, police work activity level, social interaction, perceived social support, instrumental support, hardiness total score, hardiness challenge score, hardiness commitment score, hardiness control score, and life events added over the past year. Indicator variables were used to represent the different categories. The odds ratios of experiencing traumatic stress were expressed in comparison with the reference category.

The final model includes the following variables as regression coefficients: gender, social interaction, instrumental support, trauma type "seeing abused children," trauma category "other disturbing incidents," frequency of trauma types "colleague involved in a shooting," "seeing abused children," "victims of serious traffic accidents," and "homicide

TABLE 6-5
ODDS RATIOS FOR HIGH RISK OF POSTTRAUMATIC STRESS DISORDER
MEASURED BY THE IMPACT OF EVENT SCALE (HOROWITZ ET AL., 1979) –
FINAL MODELS "INCIDENT TYPE AND FREQUENCY"

Incident Type	Model: Males (N = 70)			Model: Entire Sample (N = 115)		
	Exp(B)	*Confidence*		*Exp(B)*	*Confidence*	
(PIS1) Colleague involved in shooting	4.138*	1.065	16.071	0.466	0.108	2.021
(PIS2) Involved in shooting oneself				2.456	0.771	7.824
(PIS3) Seeing abused children	5.350*	1.048	27.306			
(PIS4) Victims of serious traffic accident	0.118*	0.017	0.819			
(PIS5) Seeing someone die						
(PIS6) Dead bodies	0.018*	0.017	0.819			
(PIS7) Severely assaulted victims						
(PIS8) Victims of homicide						
(PIS9) Other disturbing incidents	2.930	0.797	10.774	3.495**	1.413	8.644
Frequency of Incidents – Number of Times Past Year	*Exp(B)*	*Confidence*		*Exp(B)*	*Confidence*	
(PIS1A) Colleague involved in shooting				2.650*	1.015	6.918
(PIS2A) Involved in shooting oneself						
(PIS3A) Seeing abused children	1.067	0.984	1.156	1.041	0.967	1.120
(PIS4A) Victims of serious traffic accident						
(PIS5A) Seeing someone die				1.257	0.884	1.786
(PIS6A) Dead bodies						
(PIS7A) Severely assaulted victims	0.970	0.924	1.108	0.991	0.956	1.027
(PIS8A) Victims of homicide	1.769*	1.137	2.753	1.189	0.984	1.437
(PIS9A) Other disturbing incidents						
–2LL	68.600			124.505		
Change in –2LL	27.524***			32.397***		
Class table % OK	80.0			65.3		
% Predicted high risk	74.2			74.8		
Goodness of FIT	Chi – Square 8.130			Chi - Square 8.317		
(Hosmer-Lemeshow)	Significance .0421			Significance 0.305		

Significance: * p < 0.05; ** p < 0.01; *** p < 0.001

victims" over the past year. Four out of nine variables within this model showed statistical significance (see Table 6-6).

Women within this sample have a 2.502 times higher traumatic stress risk than their male counterparts (confidence interval 0.846 to 7.401, p = 0.097). Social interaction demonstrates statistical significance in general (p = 0.001). Persons who interacted with 11 to 16 persons within their social network were at a 5.083 higher risk than those who interacted with 4 to 10 persons (confidence interval 1.213 to 21.302, p = 0.026). Socializing regularly with 17 to 26 persons increases traumatic stress risk by a factor of 9.033 compared with those socializing with 4 to 10 persons in the social network (confidence interval 1.997 to 40.860, p = 0.004). For officers who interact with more than 26 persons regularly, risk decreases by a factor of 0.446 compared with those interacting with 4 to 10 persons (confidence interval 0.094 to 2.120, p = 0.310). Receiving low social support reduces risk by a factor of 0.480 compared with receiving high instrumental support (confidence interval 0.175 to 1.316, p = 0.154).

Confrontation with abused children puts an officer at a 2.542 higher risk than officers who do not have this experience (confidence interval 0.741 to 8.721, p = 0.138). Exposure to traumata within the category "other disturbing incidents" elevates traumatic stress risk by a factor of 4.489 (confidence interval 1.578 to 12.770, p = 0.005).

Every time an officer experiences a shooting involving a colleague, traumatic stress risk is increased by a factor of 3.629 (confidence interval 1.569 to 8.394, p = 0.003). The influence of frequency of seeing abused children is reflected by an odds ratio of 1.063 (confidence interval 0.972 to 1.162, p = 0.181), which is nearly 1 and therefore has minimal influence on risk. A similar result was shown for the frequency of trauma type "victims of serious traffic accidents" with an odds ratio of 1.163 (confidence interval 0.935 to 1.447, p = 0.175). The frequency of being confronted with homicide victims had a statistically significant influence on traumatic stress risk. Every time an officer is confronted with homicide victims, his traumatic stress risk increases by a factor of 1.254 (confidence interval 1.060 to 1.482, p = 0.008).

For "hardiness," as well as for the remaining variables described above, no effect could be demonstrated in the final model. The final model predicts traumatic stress risk correctly for 80.0% of all cases, which is a satisfying percentage. High risk was predicted correctly in 75.5% of all officers. The final model is summarized in Table 6-6.

TABLE 6-6
ODDS RATIOS FOR HIGH RISK OF POSTTRAUMATIC STRESS DISORDER
MEASURED BY THE IMPACT OF EVENT SCALE (HOROWITZ ET AL., 1979) –
FINAL MODELS "MEDIATING VARIABLES"

	Model: Moderator Variables (N = 115)			
Incident Type	*Exp(B)*	*Significance*	*Confidence Interval*	
(PIS3) Seeing abused children	2.542	0.138	0.741	8.721
(PIS9) Other disturbing incidents	4.489*	0.005	1.578	12.770
Frequency of Incidents – Number of Times Past Year	*Exp(B)*	*Significance*	*Confidence Interval*	
Shooting another officer	3.629**	0.003	1.569	8.394
Seeing abused children	1.063	0.181	0.972	1.162
Victims of homicide	1.163	0.175	0.935	1.447
Victims of homicide	1.254**	0.008	1.060	1.482
Moderator Variables	*Exp(B)*	*Significance*	*Confidence Interval*	
Gender (Female)	2.502	0.097	0.846	7.401
Social interactions				
4–10 persons (reference)	1.000			
11–16 persons	5.083*	0.026	1.213	21.302
17–26 persons	9.033**	0.004	1.997	40.860
> 26 persons	0.446	0.310	0.094	2.120
Instrumental support (low)	0.480	0.154	0.175	1.316
–2LL	103.215			
Change in –2LL	53.687**			
Class table % OK	80.0			
% Predicted high risk	75.5			
Goodness of FIT	Chi – Square 4.630			
(Hosmer-Lemeshow)	Significance 0.796			

Significance: * p < 0.05; ** p < 0.01; *** p < 0.001

DISCUSSION

Limitations of The Study

There are some limitations in this study. The sample size, although random and based on a 100% collection rate, is small (N = 115). Larger samples will increase reliability. No data on officers' traumatic experiences prior to commencement were available. However, screening during the selection process may minimize risk from this quarter. Officers may have experienced but not mentioned some traumatic incidents, and this could have influenced outcomes.

Although only some of the examined variables were significant predictors, others may have contributed to their risk status. More work is required to assess their potential influence. The likelihood of consistent exposure to traumatic events was higher for male participants than for female officers (see Table 6-1), but it was comparable in most types.

Trauma Type

Regression models differed between female and male participants. While the shooting of a colleague decreased stress risk in women by a factor of 0.038, it increased the risk in men by a factor of 4.422. The latter may be explained by the "ripple effect," which describes how the impact of trauma spreads out "to affect individuals on the basis of their physical or psychological association with an event or those affected, and extends risk status to others" because of cohesion within this occupational group (Paton & Smith, 1999, p. 13). Surprisingly, no effect was shown for the entire sample in terms of this trauma type. This absence of effect may be due to the contrasting nature of female and male participants in terms their experience of a shooting involving a colleague.

Confrontation with abused children elevated risk for both females and males, and particularly for female officers (odds ratio of almost 33). Brown et al. (1999) stated that female officers were more likely to be assigned to sexual offenses, and this factor raises their likelihood of suffering psychological distress from this hazard. In the present sample, the number of females and males who did experience exposure to abused children as one form of sexual offense was almost similar, but the number of males was even higher (60% vs. 72.9%). Hence the quantity of assignments is not an explanation within this sample. In general, women are more likely to be victims of sexual offenses. Therefore, retraumatization or a stronger identification with the victim may be an interpretation.

Traumatic stress risk is increased by a factor of 15.56 in terms of confrontation with victims of homicide for male participants, whereas no effect was shown for female officers. The biggest contributor to risk in female officers was represented by "other disturbing incidents" with an odds ratio of 35. This category includes several traumata; hence, it is not possible to interpret this result specifically. It is interesting that this trauma category did not show an effect for male participants. For the entire sample, this hazard increases traumatic stress risk by a factor of 2.44.

Trauma Type and Frequency

The final model for male officers included four of seven statistically significant coefficients, whereas the final model for the entire sample contains only two out of eight significant regression coefficients. Statistically significant coefficients differ between the two models, even if five coefficients are included in both. The trauma type "colleague involved in a shooting" increased stress risk in male officers by a factor of 4.138, whereas it showed a decreasing influence by 0.466 in the entire sample, even if not statistically significant. This difference may be due to the fact that female participants showed a decreasing risk of PTSD from the impact of shootings involving a colleague. Confrontation with victims of serious traffic accidents puts male officers under a 5.350 higher risk than officers without this exposure. It is worth noting that this type did not show an effect in the final model of male participants for the influence of type of traumatic incident. It did not demonstrate an influence for women or for the entire sample either.

Seeing dead bodies decreased stress risk in male participants by a factor of 0.118. A similar result was shown for the final model "trauma type." The reduced risk calculated in this regression analysis may be due to adaptation. The principle here may be "the more you see it, the less it bothers you." Another explanation could be that seeing dead bodies includes natural death; hence, it may be acceptable compared with violent acts like homicide. "Other disturbing incidents" showed a statistically significant influence in the entire sample and increased traumatic stress risk by a factor of 3.945. An effect also was shown for male participants, even without statistical significance.

While the trauma type "colleague involved in shooting" increased the risk of PTSD in male officers, its frequency had an elevating effect in the entire sample (odds ratio 2.650), which means that every occurrence of this type has an impact on the officers by a factor of 2.650. The frequency of the trauma type "seeing abused children" had a negligible effect (odds ratio of 1.067/1.041), even without statistic significance. The trauma type itself had a great impact on the officers' risk in the final models of the influence of type of traumatic incident. Therefore, traumatic stress risk differs between officers who experienced a confrontation with abused children compared with officers who have not been exposed, but the frequency of this type of trauma does not have an influence.

A similar result applied for the frequency of the trauma type "severely assaulted victims" with odds ratios of 0.970 or 0.991. The frequency of exposure to "homicide victims" showed an effect of 1.769 in male officers and a lower influence of 1.189 in the entire sample. In comparison with the odds ratio of 15.560 in the final model "trauma type" of male officers, the effect of the frequency was slight. Hence, the occurrence itself has a bigger impact than the frequency of being exposed to homicide victims.

Mediating Variables

The model's "mediating variables" include five out of eleven coefficients that show statistic significance in the present sample. Two trauma types have an impact within this model. "Seeing abused children" influences traumatic stress risk by a factor of 2.542, with is indeed without statistic significance. It did show an effect in an earlier model. The trauma category "other disturbing incidents" increased stress risk by a factor of 4.489. This result is higher than the coefficients in model "trauma type" and "trauma type and frequency" for the entire sample. The interaction of the included variables may be an explanation for this finding. Every regression model is a network of variables; hence they are connected and depend on each other.

Four types of trauma frequencies increased traumatic stress risk. A shooting of another officer influences the risk by a factor of 3.629 within this regression model. This odds ratio is a higher than that in the final model "trauma type and frequency" for the entire sample; nevertheless, it can be seen as comparable. The odds ratios of trauma frequency for the types of incident "seeing abused children" and "victims of serious traffic accidents" are nearly 1 and, therefore, show no significant effect. While the frequency of exposure to victims of serious traffic accidents has not been included before, the result in terms of the trauma frequency "seeing abused children" is consistent with the findings before. The fourth coefficient is the frequency of exposure to "victims of homicide" with an odds ratio of 1.254. This ratio is comparable to the impact in the final model "trauma type and frequency" for the entire sample, as well as for male officers.

Concerning the mediating variables, three showed an effect. Gender increased traumatic stress risk. Being female increased risk by a factor of 2.505. This result confirms the findings of Davis and Breslau (1998), Halligan and Yehuda (2000), and Maercker (1997). The variable "social interaction" influenced stress risk significantly. Three different aspects of social interaction were influential here. Interaction with 11 to 16 persons regularly increased the risk by a factor of 5.083; having a social network of 17 to 26 persons increased risk by a factor of 9.033. This effect is significant. A possible explanation is connected to the occupational culture of police officers. The image of a strong male, especially within a male-dominated police occupation, is reflected in components like having no fear, no pain, no helplessness, no grief, and no trauma (Pieper & Maercker,1999, p. 223). To be strong and indestructible represents a common stereotype for this occupation. Hence, as the number of people one interacts with grows, the greater is the pressure to avoid emotions and feelings, but the harder it is to maintain, because people usually have a sense for emotions in persons with whom they are interacting. Of greater interest is the influence of interaction with more than 26 persons on a regular basis, which decreases risk by 0.480.

The third mediating variable investigated was social support. Low social instrumental support decreased the risk by a factor of 0.480 (without statistic significance). This finding may be interpreted in the same way as the results for social interaction. The need of instrumental support is linked to the admission of need for help. Helplessness is equivalent to losing control, an important predictor of adverse stress reactions. As described before, stereotypical aspects of police culture hinder a use of instrumental social support as a source for resistance and coping. Therefore, low instrumental support acts to maintain the self-image of invulnerability better than receiving visible objective support; hence, it is less threatening to an officer's self-esteem.

CONCLUSION

Several factors predict high traumatic stress risk in the present sample of 115 police officers. These factors were analyzed in terms of type and frequency of the prescribed trauma. Even though the random sample of police officers employed in the study is small, it provides baseline information for future work in this area. While some trauma types, frequencies, and mediating variables did not affect stress risk, the limitations of the present study mean that additional longitudinal research into their influence is required. For example, the trauma type "police shootings," which appears to be one of the most highly rated police traumas, was experienced by only 14.8% of our sample within the past year. For those factors that did predict officers' traumatic stress risk, additional work on moderating variables that may either increase or decrease this risk is required. Prevention and intervention programs developed by police organizations may be helpful in completing such a task. Police work is a psychologically dangerous occupation, and there is much to be accomplished through research to make it safer.

REFERENCES

Allen, J. G. (1995). *Coping with Trauma: A Guide to Self-understanding.* Washington, DC: American Psychiatric Press.

American Psychiatric Association. (1994). *Diagnostic and Statistical Manual of Mental Disorders* (4th ed.). Washington: APA.

Bartone, P. T. (1995). *A Short Hardiness Scale.* Paper presented at the annual convention of the American Psychological Society, New York.

Brewin, C. R., Andrews, B., & Valentine, J. D. (2000). Meta-analysis of risk factors for posttraumatic stress disorder in trauma-exposed adults. *Journal of Consulting and Clinical Psychology, 68,* 748–766.

Brown, J., Fielding, J., & Grover, J. (1999). Distinguishing traumatic, vicarious and routine operational stressor exposure and attendant adverse consequences in a sample of police officers. *Work & Stress, 13*(4), 312–325.

Davis, G. C., & Breslau, N. (1998). Are women at greater risk for PTSD than men? *Psychiatric Times, 7.* Retrieved January 25, 2003, from http://www.psychiatrictimes.com/p980765.html

Green, B. L. (1994). Psychosocial research in traumatic stress: An update. *Journal of Traumatic Stress, 7,* 341–362.

Halligan, S. L., & Yehuda, R. (2000). Risk factors for PTSD. *PTSD Research Quarterly, 11*(3), 1–8.

Horowitz, M. J., Wilner, N., & Alvarez, W. (1979). Impact of Event Scale: A measure of subjective stress. *Psychosomatic Medicine, 41,* 209–218.

Kessler, R. C., Sonnega, A., Bromet, E., Hughes, M., & Nelson, C. B. (1995). Posttraumatic stress disorder in the National Comorbidity Survey. *Archives of General Psychiatry, 52,* 1048–1060.

Kobasa, S. (1979). Stressful life events, personality, and health: An inquiry into hardiness. *Journal of Personality and Social Psychology, 37,* 1–11.

Lucas, M. G. (2000). Notfallpsychologie: Grundlagen, Konzepte, Fortbildungsangebote. Emergency psychology: Fundamentals, concepts, offers for further training. In J. Schatte & B. Weißgerber (Eds.), *Psychologische Vor- und Nachsorge für Beschäftigte von Berufsgruppen, die mit Notfallsituationen konfrontiert sind* (pp. 13–23). Dortmund, Germany: Bundesanstalt für Arbeitsschutz und Arbeitsmedizin.

Maercker, A. (Ed.) (1997). Therapie der posttraumatischen Belastungsstörungen. *Therapy of Posttraumatic Stress Disorders.* Berlin: Springer.

Paton, D., & Smith, L. (1999). Assessment, conceptual and methodological issues in researching traumatic stress in police officers. In J. M. Violanti & D. Paton (Eds.), *Police Trauma: Psychological Aftermath of Civilian Combat* (pp. 13–24). Springfield, IL: Charles C Thomas.

Pieper, G., & Maercker, A. (1999). Männlichkeit und Verleugnung von Hilfsbedürftigkeit nach berufsbedingten Traumata (Polizei, Feuerwehr, Rettungspersonal) Masculinity and avoidance of help-seeking after job-related trauma (Police, Firefighters, Rescue Teams). *Verhaltenstherapie, 9,* 222–229.

Sundin, E. C., & Horowitz, M. J. (2002). Impact of Event Scale: Psychometric properties. *British Journal of Psychiatry, 180,* 205–209.

Chapter 7

RISK FACTORS IN EMERGENCY RESPONDERS

DOUGLAS PATON AND GREG HANNAN

INTRODUCTION

The careers of members of several professions (e.g., law enforcement, fire and rescue services) will be punctuated by periodic exposure to complex disasters. For these professions, stress risk management commences with the identification of the event characteristics and demands (Davies & Walters, 1998; Moran & Colless, 1995; Paton, 1997) and organizational and managerial practices that constitute the hazards associated with traumatic stress risk (Alexander & Wells, 1991; Eränen, Millar, & Paton, 1999; Gist & Woodall, 2000; Hart & Wearing, 1995; Paton, Smith, Ramsay, & Akande, 1999). Although discussion of adverse reactions has dominated the stress literature, exposure to these risk factors need not necessarily have negative consequences. It is becoming increasingly evident that disaster duties can result in positive outcomes for response personnel (Anderson, Christensen, & Petersen, 1991; Alexander & Wells, 1991; Moran, 1999; Moran & Colless, 1995; Paton, Violanti, & Smith, 2003).

The complexity of the demands encountered can provide officers with opportunities to exercise professional skills to achieve highly meaningful outcomes (e.g., saving life) in a manner rarely possible in routine contexts. Characteristics such as teamwork, a sense of group identity, and the suspension of bureaucracy and politics have also been implicated in this context. Positive outcomes have also been associated with incident experiences that result in a sense of exhilaration, a sense of appreciation of life, and a sense of control over significant adverse events. Consequently, it is important to consider how hazard exposure leads to both positive and negative outcomes.

Comprehensive stress risk management also requires understanding how emergency responders' involvement in disasters changes over time. Emergencies are experienced as a series of phases (see Schmuckler, ch. 2): alarm or warning and mobilization, the response, and the subsequent reintegration into routine work. This chapter discusses these phases and their implications for stress risk.

RISK FACTORS DURING THE ALARM AND MOBILIZATION PHASE

The alarm phase describes the period of comprehending and adjusting to the occurrence of a disaster. The demands that typify this phase include, for example, accessing intelligence about the disaster, differentiating fact from inference, and making sense of information about what is, by definition, a nonroutine event. However, emergency planning and training that assists officers to impose a sense of coherence on atypical events increases the likelihood of mobilization activities promoting positive outcomes (Paton, Johnston, & Houghton, 1998; Paton & Jackson, 2002). For those in command roles, stress risk is also influenced by demands associated with formulating and adapting plans to fit situational demands and identifying and deploying the resources required for incident management. Because facilitating positive outcomes from exposure to this risk factor is a function of the ability to extract salient cues that assist their adapting plans and response actions to fit situational demands, officers' situational awareness is essential to understanding mobilization stress risk.

Situation awareness (SA) has been defined as both a process (sometimes referred to as "situation assessment") and a state characterized by a sound comprehension of events and details associated with those events (Salas, Prince, Baker, & Shestra, 1995; Sarter & Woods, 1991). Endsley (1988) proposes three levels of SA: perception of elements relevant to events; comprehension of those elements in relation to the events; and projection of that comprehension into the future (short term). Sarter and Woods (1991) also emphasize the importance of the temporal nature of SA, a reasonable proposition given that events take place in a volume of time and space and that the process of developing and maintaining it is a dynamic one.

During mobilization, officers have limited opportunities to develop SA since information about a specific event will be sketchy and uncorroborated. This may increase stress vulnerability at this stage, but could be offset by training and experience on the specific emergency types around which SA could be developed. This underlines the importance of adopting an all-hazards approach to design training that facilitates an adaptive response capability (Paton, 1994). The use of knowledge gained from previous scenarios and missions would thus be available during mobilization to develop initial team SA and to formulate alternative hypotheses about the nature of the event and possible responses to it.

During the alarm and mobilization phase, another significant risk factor is the timing of deployment. The likelihood of negative outcomes arising from exposure to this risk factor is higher when emergency call-outs result in officers being deployed before a full appreciation of the nature or implications of a disaster is known. For example, officers deployed immediately to the site of the Lockerbie disaster found it difficult to comprehend the carnage and death encountered (Mitchell, 1991). While performing similar duties in a similar environment, officers deployed once the nature and probable cause of the event were known (a terrorist bombing) reported significantly lower levels of stress. Being able to define their situation as a criminal investigation allowed them to apply their professional expertise (i.e., dealing with body parts as an evidence gathering procedure) in a more meaningful manner.

While a long mobilization or warning period may reduce stress risk associated with event comprehension, risk during this period can be influenced by other factors. Because they are action-orientated, emergency responders are motivated to respond quickly. However, for prolonged, complex events, the time required to formulate response plans, resource needs, and deployment strategies can result in delays that, unless filled with constructive activities (e.g., checking equipment, planning response tactics, generating realistic response expectations), can constitute a mobilization stressor (Paton, 1994).

Mobilization stress risk is greater if personnel are responding at the end of a shift or if they are affected by transient factors such as illness or occupational stress (Flin, 1996). The nature and level of routine work demands prior to deployment and family issues also constitute risk factors (Flin, 1996; Hart & Wearing, 1995; Shakespeare-Finch, Paton & Violanti,

2003). The personal and transient nature of these factors renders them difficult to control or manage. However, risk management programs that focus on enhancing officers' awareness of these limiting factors, their implications for performance, and the need to adopt appropriate management strategies (e.g., increased teamwork, adequate rest breaks, rotation of personnel) can mitigate adverse consequences.

RISK FACTORS DURING THE RESPONSE PHASE

During the response phase, risk factors can emanate from incident characteristics, role stress, and organizational and management practices. For example, those responding to the devastation associated with a large earthquake or the aftermath of a terrorist bombing encounter death and human suffering, hazards from disrupted sewerage systems, unstable buildings, increased health risks, and separation from their families. Event causation is a risk factor, with those resulting from acts of human omission (e.g., building collapse from poor workmanship) or commission (e.g., terrorist bombing) being particularly likely to trigger negative outcomes.

Uncertainty about, for example, the duration of a threat, its recurrence, or additional threats (e.g., earthquake aftershocks, further building collapse) heightens the risk of experiencing negative reactions. Consequently, personal danger (e.g., working in a damaged building, exposure to contaminated blood products or infectious diseases) and the need to safeguard members of the public from threatening circumstances are prominent stressors. In regard to sources of danger, events that pose unseen threats (e.g., highly toxic chemical, biological, or radiation hazards), by making it more difficult for officers to take protective actions, increase stress vulnerability. Environmental factors such as heat, noise, or poor visibility increase stress and create a similar risk (Vrij, van der Steen, & Koppelaar, 1994), as do the sights, sounds and, especially, the smells associated with adverse events (Paton, Cox, & Andrew, 1989; Taylor & Frazer, 1982).

Stress risk is particularly pronounced when duties involve the recovery and identification of bodies and human remains. Training and experience of handling body remains lessens stress in those exposed to this activity for prolonged periods, but less so for those exposed for relatively short periods (Alexander & Wells, 1991; Deahl et al., 1994; Thompson,

1993). This difference is possibly related to the time it takes to invoke particular coping strategies such as imagery. Although imagery can be an effective coping strategy during body recovery duties, it can constitute a source of stress following the termination of these duties as personnel review their actions and thoughts (Paton et al., 1989; Taylor & Frazer, 1982). Stress risk is also influenced by media reporting. Sensationalizing, misreporting, or generating rumors about the response and/or how it was managed are prominent stressors in this context.

Family and other associations with the location of a disaster or those directly affected are a risk factors. When colleagues are injured, killed, or experience significant loss, a process of identification with them (e.g., from a sense of shared fate from working in the same agency, performing the same role) influences stress vulnerability.

In complex, prolonged incidents, operational personnel can find their roles changing frequently (e.g., from rescuing someone from a collapsed building, to crowd control, to comforting relatives, to talking to the media), increasing both the demands made upon them and opportunities to question the validity and appropriateness of their actions. Insufficient, inadequate, or inappropriate resources to perform response tasks can fuel a sense of inadequacy and increase stress vulnerability (Paton, 1994).

Stress risk is influenced by the opportunities afforded for effective action by the characteristics of a specific disaster. When event characteristics limit such opportunities, negative outcomes are likely if beliefs about a perceived response failure are internalized rather than being attributed, more accurately, to environmental constraints beyond an officer's control (MacLeod & Paton, 1999; Paton & Stephens, 1996). The ensuing reaction has been labeled "performance guilt" (Raphael, 1986) or "responsibility trauma" (Williams, 1993). To counter this, training should focus on the development of realistic outcome expectations, the ability to differentiate personal and situational constraints, and interpretive processes that review experiences as learning opportunities that enhance future understanding and performance (MacLeod & Paton, 1999; Paton, 1994).

Emergency response is typically a team activity. Stress risk is influenced by coordination problems and role ambiguity (Paton, 1994). However, training in team skills and extensive joint planning and teamwork activity involving team members can moderate adverse reactions (Brannick, Salas, & Prince, 1997; Flin, 1996; Paton et al., 1999a; Pollock et al., 2003; Salas et al., 1999), with good information sharing being a prominent determinant of this improvement. In effective teams, members provide more unprompted information, increasing a capability for proactive response management through better tactical decision making and resource allocation (Entin & Serfaty, 1999). For this to occur effectively, team members must share a "team mental model" (also referred to as a "shared mental model," Salas et al., 1995), specifically relating to the goal-related information required by decision makers at critical periods (Cooke et al., 2000). As the level of teamwork and planning activity increases, officers develop progressively similar mental models of response environments and the roles and tasks to be performed within them. This, in turn, increases implicit information sharing during high workload periods, enhancing team performance (Paton & Jackson, 2002; Stout et al., 1999) and increasing the likelihood of team members' experiencing positive outcomes.

The point needs to be made, however, that the capacity of team members to develop their own mental models (SA) and then share information to develop a "shared mental model" of an event is contingent on several significant factors, particularly individual differences in the cognitive capacities of team members and their ability to communicate in efficient, constructive, and meaningful ways. Teams that lack these skills may be more vulnerable to stress and therefore less likely to experience positive outcomes.

Stress risk is influenced by other social-cognitive processes. Although emergency personnel may possess the technical skill and knowledge to respond, the operational mental models derived from routine experience that are essential to response planning and organizing action may be unable to impose coherence upon atypical and complex emergency situations (Dunning, 2003; Paton, 1994). Inappropriate assumptions regarding operating conditions, performance expectations, roles, and tasks and the consequent need for rapid situational reframing significantly increase stress vulnerability. However, training that facilitates officers' ability to impose meaning and coherence on atypical events can facilitate positive outcomes; enhance performance, control, and adaptability across a range of incidents; and hasten recovery (Alexander & Wells, 1991; Driskell & Salas, 1996; Dunning, 2003; Paton, 1994; Paton & Jackson, 2002).

To facilitate the development of these mental models, simulations are increasingly being used as training resources. Simulations afford opportunities for officers to develop, practice, and review technical, management, and team skills under realistic circumstances; construct realistic performance expectations; practice dealing with high pressure situations in a safe and supportive environment; increase awareness of stress reactions; and rehearse strategies to minimize negative reactions (Crego & Spinks, 1997; Paton & Jackson, 2002). They also provide a medium through which officers can receive feedback on their performance, define areas for development, and identify organizational factors that act as response risk factors (e.g., inadequate delegation or decision systems).

For the development of these more sophisticated psychological structures, two things are required. One involves the systematic analysis of emergency roles, tasks, and responsibilities to define the skills and knowledge required for effective response across a range of incidents. The second concerns the design of simulations to reconcile disaster characteristics and response demands (e.g., scale of damage, multiagency operations, rapid role change) with response practices (Flin, 1996; Paton, 1994; Paton & Jackson, 2002). Simulation should address, for example, the identification of risk factors and their consequences for disaster stress (such as those discussed above); the translation of plans into action and adaptation of them to cater for events differing in type, scale, or complexity; team processes and management; delegation of authority; communication, creative problem solving and decision-making under conditions of uncertainty; and multiagency response management (Paton et al., 1998; Paton et al., 1999a; Pollock et al., 2003).

Greater than expected and/or unexpected responsibility is a stressor. Officers may find themselves making decisions normally made by other or more senior personnel, often with incomplete or inaccurate information about an evolving incident. They may be working in a context of changing and possibly ambiguous goals involving members of several agencies, and they may be under considerable time pressure. Factors that influence stress risk in this context are communication, situational awareness, decision-making processes, the time available, and the level of risk associated with a decision.

Information Management and Situational Awareness

Stress risk is influenced by the availability of information for decision making and officers' ability to render it meaningful in regard to the situational demands encountered. While some problems will reflect hazard activity (e.g., damage to communication infrastructure), the key issue here is the adequacy of information management procedures (Paton & Flin 1999). Effective emergency communication requires that information needs are anticipated and defined, that networks with information providers and recipients are organized, and that officers have the capability to provide, access, collate, interpret ,and disseminate information compatible with decision needs and systems that are established (Paton et al., 1999a).

These processes and systems are central to officers' developing and maintaining situation awareness and shared mental models within and across teams during an emergency response. Salas et al. (1995) point out that SA is dynamic and needs to be continually updated. The availability of information and the methods of processing, interpreting, and disseminating that information are critical to SA of individuals and teams and, therefore, key predictors of stress vulnerability in officers. Before discussion of methods of information transfer and their role in the development of shared mental models, it is worth noting that the type of large-scale emergency implied in this discussion involves the coordination of several emergency teams with different goals, equipment, and methods. These scenarios take SA to a new level of complexity, from an individual team member's SA, to a shared mental model within a team, to shared models across teams who are often working at different physical locations on different aspects of the emergency.

In these situations, information flow and the ability to access it are critical determinants of the how efficiently and effectively teams can develop and maintain SA when responding to complex and possibly escalating events. Salas et al. (1995) stress the importance of information-seeking skills (and how to elicit information from other sources, in particular) within individual team members as an important base skill in developing shared mental models.

At a team level communication behaviors have been indicated as important factors in acquiring and maintaining accurate shared mental models. Artman (1999) found that the process of team members' "thinking aloud" and regularly discussing information received in a control environment produced better shared models than in environments where team members did not engage in these behaviors. Command structure also influences team effectiveness. Artman (1999, 2000) found that serial (or hierarchical) structures produce more efficient and sound shared mental models in both civilian and military command environments. Artman's explanation for this is that in serially structured environments the team members are obliged to share information and therefore hold a greater percentage of shared information. The downside of this is that in high workload situations there is the risk of overload.

On the basis of the above arguments, training in methods to acquire and maintain SA in these complex emergency situations needs to be modified beyond existing approaches (Salas et al., 1995). Travillian, Volpe, Cannon-Bowers, and Salas (1993) argue that cross training of team members in each other's roles improves team performance. Consequently, cross training teams in the role and methods of other emergency teams could enhance the SA and shared mental models of the emergency and facilitate a more efficient and productive flow of information between teams or to a coordination command center (Artman, 1999; Marks, Sabella, Burke, & Zaccaro, 2002).

Decision Making

For trained personnel, the high demands associated with emergency response can enhance decision-making performance by increasing alertness, reactions, and energy and by accelerating thinking skills (Flin, 1996). These effects facilitate officers' ability to react to atypical and emergent demands and to take decisions under pressure. However, emergency responders faced with substantial physical and time pressures, particularly if working for prolonged periods under complex, threatening circumstances, risk developing "counter disaster syndrome" (Raphael, 1986), a state in which they feel that response effectiveness hinges on their personal involvement. The ensuing combination of fatigue and continued exposure to response demands can, as a consequence of officers' experiencing "tunnel vision," failure to prioritize, "freezing," and loss of concentration, detrimentally affect decision making (Flin, 1996) and increase stress vulnerability.

The decision-making process used also influences stress risk. One process describes analytical decision making, through which the individual or team consider alternative courses of action and select the best option. This contrasts with intuitive or naturalistic decision making, through which the person recognizes the type of situation encountered and, from previous experience, selects an appropriate course of action (Flin et al., 1997). Naturalistic decision style has been observed in fire fighting (Burke & Hendry, 1997), emergency evacuation (Flin, Slaven, & Stewart, 1996), and aviation (Orasanu, 1997) incidents characterized by substantial time pressure and high risk. Klein (1996) has argued that the naturalistic decision style is less affected by stress than by the more intellectually demanding analytical approach. However, the latter remains the most appropriate style for those involved in strategic decision making (Flin, 1996). When time pressures and risk are high, success in naturalistic decision making is a function of the ability to match current and prior situations. Decision effectiveness will be enhanced with more options to match. This ability can be developed through experience or simulation.

Management Context

Stress vulnerability is heightened by inadequate disaster management procedures (Alexander & Wells, 1991; Flin, 1996; Gist & Woodall, 2000; Hart & Wearing, 1995; Paton & Flin, 1999; Paton, 1997). Persistent use of established operational and decision procedures (even when responding to different and urgent crisis demands), internal conflicts regarding responsibility, and a desire to protect the organization from criticism or blame complicate the response process. The adoption of autonomous emergency management systems, a consultative leadership style, and practices that ensure that role and task assignments reflect incident demands can ameliorate stress (Alexander & Wells, 1991; Gist & Woodall, 2000; Paton, 1994).

These problems are compounded when operating in multiagency settings (Paton & Flin, 1999; Paton, et al., 1999a; Paton et al., 1998). Inadequate coordination increases conflict between agencies, results in a blurring of roles and responsibilities, and fuels frustration and feelings of inadequacy and helplessness (Paton, 1994). Facilitating positive outcomes from exposure to this risk factor requires liaison mechanisms to integrate the respective roles and operating practices of responding agencies.

RISK FACTORS DURING THE LETDOWN AND REINTEGRATION PHASE

From a risk-management perspective, reintegration and recovery management are important in two respects. Whereas exposure to risk factors during response has increased stress vulnerability, stress management during reintegration should focus on both the positive management of the emotional correlates of officers' experience and on assisting them to interpret the event and experiences in meaningful and coherent ways. Support practices designed to assist positive resolution are discussed elsewhere (Dunning, 1999; Calhoun & Tedeschi, 2000; Paton & Stephens, 1996).

Termination of involvement in disaster response does not mean that stress risk is eliminated. The period of transition from working in the high-demand disaster context back into routine work and family life poses a unique set of risk factors. During this stage, the officers' process of working through and making sense of their feelings (and those of others) represents a risk factor, but not necessarily one that only reflects the experience of negative emotional reactions from their involvement. Positive interpretations during response can become a risk factor for negative reactions during reintegration. For example, personnel may experience feelings of loss as they move out of an action phase characterized by high levels of perceived personal and/or professional performance, or negative feelings may be intensified as officers return to "business as usual" and readjust to family life (Paton & Stephens, 1996; Shakespeare-Finch et al., 2003). In addition to the stress emanating from their own experience, organizational factors (e.g., shift work, organizational climate) are prominent family risk factors (Eränen et al., 1999; Shakespeare-Finch et al., 2003). This fact signals the need for organizational planning to include stress management for family members (Shakespeare-Finch et al., 2003).

For officers, readjusting to normal routines, dealing with paperwork, catching up with any backlog of work, and dealing with any legal correlates of the response constitute significant demands. However, the psychological implications of these demands are a function of both the officers' ability to render their experiences meaningful and the extent to which senior officers possess the capability and/or willingness to manage the recovery and reintegration phase in a manner that sustains or facilitates adaptation (Alexander & Wells, 1991; Paton & Violanti, 1996; Violanti & Paton, 1999). For example, a cultural predisposition within an emergency organization to suppress emotional disclosure, focus on attributing blame, or to minimize the significance of peoples' reactions or feelings can undermine support provision, heighten stress vulnerability, and extend performance deficits (Paton & Stephens, 1996; MacLeod & Paton, 1999).

The likelihood of positive reintegration is heightened if senior managers and their officers work collectively to reconcile the personal impact of the event with the process of returning to work. Senior officers also can facilitate this process by helping personnel appreciate that they performed to the best of their ability, realistically review their experiences relative to situational constraints on performance, understand that little could have been done differently under the circumstances, reduce inappropriate feelings of guilt and responsibility, learn about their reactions, and provide accurate information about what happened and about future issues (e.g., inquests, funerals, memorial services) (Alexander & Wells, 1991; MacLeod & Paton, 1999; Paton, 1997). The provision of information from a credible source helps to moderate stress associated with rumors and media reports that could otherwise create additional problems for officers and their families. Senior officers can also facilitate the positive resolution of disaster experience by assisting staff in the identification of the strengths that helped them deal with the emergency response and building upon this experience to plan how future incidents could be dealt with more effectively. However, the fact that these activities can constitute a source of stress for senior officers should be acknowledged, and support resources should be provided for them accordingly. This process can be used to enhance the knowledge base of teams and team members and to assist teams in the clarification of their mental models, not only of the event and the response to it, but also of the processes they went through during the emergency response. It can be argued that such a process would enhance team responses and SA during future mobilization and response phases.

At a more general level, risk-management programs should review the climate of relationships between managers and staff and determine its implications for support and recovery (Johnston & Paton, 2003; Paton, 1997). In the longer term, such analyses can contribute to organizational development programs through, for example, identifying response constraints within organizational systems (e.g., lack of policy and procedures for managing critical incident stress, inadequate reintegration and recovery procedures and capabilities). This information can be used both to promote future response effectiveness and to develop and maintain an organizational climate that facilitates stress resilience.

Returning to normal routines and duties is therapeutic. This helps officers put their experience into perspective, assists them to regain a sense of control, and increases access to social support resources and opportunities for discussion with others who were involved. However, the risk of experiencing adverse reactions is influenced by the temporary diminution of cognitive capabilities associated with intense emergency work. Reintegration should thus be planned and gradual to ensure that officers do not attempt to take on too much too soon, and that they take care when, for example, driving or making complex decisions.

Several group factors and the quality of the social relationships prevailing during this period affect stress risk during reintegration (Gist & Woodall, 2000; MacLeod & Paton, 1999; Paton & Stephens, 1996). Exposure to others' perspectives, experiences, and problems in regard to the incident, its causes, and the response can heighten stress vulnerability, as can rumination about poor outcomes or imagining positive outcomes contrary to those that actually occurred (MacLeod, 2000). Consequently, risk management programs should include social and peer support resources (Paton, 1994; Paton, 1997; Williams, 1993) and the promotion of cohesiveness.

Group cohesion represents a risk factor because it interacts with the manner in which officers share the experience of adversity and develop a sense of shared fate and similar affective reactions (Paton & Stephens, 1996). Cohesion can increase stress vulnerability when the response is perceived as being less effective than might have been anticipated. Under these conditions, officers may find it difficult to perceive the positive characteristics in the group necessary to maintain a positive group identity. If this happens, support networks may breakdown, a negative group social identity may develop (Paton & Stephens, 1996; Solomon & Smith, 1994), and stress vulnerability is increased. The positive benefits of cohesion are facilitated by organizational climates and managerial practices that acknowledge and legitimize emotional expression, promote self-help activities, involve realistic interpretation of circumstances, actively differentiate personal and situational response factors, and facilitate imposing coherence on atypical events by encouraging the interpretation of professional experience as learning opportunities that facilitate personal and professional growth (Dunning, 1999; Gist & Woodall, 2000; Lyons, Mickelson, Sullivan, & Coyne, 1998; MacLeod & Paton, 1999; Park, 1998; Paton & Stephens, 1996; Violanti & Paton, 1999).

CONCLUSION

Although far from comprehensive, the above discussion illustrates the diverse web of factors capable of influencing stress risk in emergency responders. Armed with this knowledge, organizations can develop appropriate mitigation strategies, including training for team coordination, information-seeking and sharing skills, and individual and team situation assessment skills. The question of officer selection also should be addressed because many of these skills are complex and difficult to master in high pressure, time-critical environments (see Dunning, ch. 3).

The manner in which emergency responders assimilate positive outcomes and resolve adverse outcomes associated with disaster work influences their future stress risk. Consequently, stress risk management should be a continuous process, and one that is accommodated within the fabric of organizational activity rather than being restricted only to the provision of support or remedial services following termination of involvement in a specific event. Although the phases discussed above were dealt with sequentially here, they should be considered holistically, with the reintegration phase from any given event acting as the foundation for the mobilization phase for the next event.

Disaster stress management programs should be developed from a comprehensive analysis of the incident, operational and organizational demands that constitute stressors during the mobilization, and response and reintegration phases. Training and simulation should be designed to promote predictability, control, and adaptability, and to ensure that operational mental models promote stress resilience by increasing a capability to impose coherence and meaning upon atypical duties. Identifying the operational, personal, and organizational determinants of positive adaptation can contribute significantly to the development of selection, training, and operational practices that promote stress resilience and psychological growth.

REFERENCES

Alexander, D. A., & Wells, A. (1991). Reactions of police officers to body handling after a major disaster: A before and after comparison. *British Journal of Psychiatry, 159,* 517–555.

Andersen, H. S., Christensen, A. K., & Petersen, G. O. (1991). Post-traumatic stress reactions amongst rescue workers after a major rail accident. *Anxiety Research, 4,* 245–251.

Artman, H. (1999). Situation awareness and co-operation within and between hierarchical units in dynamic decision making. *Ergonomics, 42,* 1404–1417.

Artman, H. (2000). Team situation assessment and information distribution. *Ergonomics, 43,* 1111–1128.

Brannick, M., Salas, E., & Prince, C. (Eds.). (1997). *Team Performance, Assessment and Measurement.* Mahwah, NJ: Lawrence Erlbaum.

Burke, E., & Hendry, C. (1997). Decision making on the London incident ground: An exploratory study. *Journal of Managerial Psychology, 12,* 40–47.

Calhoun, L. G. & Tedeschi, R. G. (2000) Early posttraumatic stress interventions: Facilitating possibilities for growth. In J.M. Violanti, D. Paton, & C. Dunning (Eds.), *Posttraumatic Stress Intervention: Challenges, Issues and Perspectives.* (pp. 135–152.). Springfield, IL: Charles C Thomas.

Cooke, N. J., Salas, E., Cannon-Bowers, J. A., & Stout, R. J. (2000). Measuring team knowledge. *Human Factors, 42,* 151–173.

Crego, J., & Spinks, T. (1997). Critical incident management simulation. In R. Flin, E. Salas, M. Strub, & L. Martin (Eds.), *Decision Making Under Stress* (pp. 85–94). Aldershot: Ashgate.

Davies, H., & Walters, M. (1998). Do all crises have to become disasters? Risk and risk mitigation. *Disaster Prevention and Management, 7,* 396–400.

Deahl, M. P., Gillham, A. B., Thomas, J., Searle, M. M., & Srinivasan, M. (1994). Psychological sequelae following the Gulf War: Factors associated with subsequent morbidity and the effectiveness of psychological debriefing. *British Journal of Psychiatry, 165,* 60–65.

Doepal, D. (1991). Crisis management: The psychological dimension. *Industrial Crisis Quarterly, 5,* 177–188.

Driskell, J., & Salas, E. (1996). *Stress and Human Performance.* Hillsdale, NJ: Lawrence Erlbaum.

Dunning, C. (1999). Post-intervention strategies to reduce police trauma: A paradigm shift. In J. M. Violanti & D. Paton (Eds.), *Police Trauma: Psychological Aftermath of Civilian Combat* (pp. 269–292). Springfield, IL: Charles C Thomas.

Dunning, C. (2003). Sense of coherence in managing trauma workers. In D. Paton, J. M. Violanti, & L. M. Smith (Eds.), *Promoting Capabilities to Manage Posttraumatic Stress: Perspectives on Resilience* (pp. 119–135). Springfield, IL: Charles C Thomas.

Endsley, M. R. (1988). Design and evaluation for situation awareness enhancement. In *Proceedings of the Human Factors Society 32nd Annual Meeting* (pp. 97–101). Santa Monica, CA: Human Factors Society.

Entin, E. E., & Serfaty, D. (1999). Adaptive team coordination. *Human Factors, 41,* 312–325.

Eränen, L., Millar, M., & Paton, D. (1999, June). *Organisational recovery from disaster: Traumatic response within voluntary disaster workers.* Paper presented at the International Society for Stress Studies Conference, Istanbul, Turkey.

Flin, R. (1996). *Sitting in the Hot Seat: Leaders and Teams for Critical Incident Management.* Chichester: Wiley.

Flin, R., Salas, E., Strub, M., & Martin, L. (Eds.) (1997). *Decision Making under Stress.* Aldershot: Ashgate.

Flin, R., Slaven, G., & Stewart, K. (1996). Emergency decision making in the offshore oil and gas industry. *Human Factors, 38,* 262–287.

Flin, R., Wynn, V., Ellis, A., & Skriver, J. (1998). *The effects of sleep loss on commanders' decision making: A literature review* (Report to Defence Evaluation Research Agency, Project No. CHS7381). Farnborough: Centre for Human Sciences.

Gist, R., & Woodall, J. (2000). There are no simple solutions to complex problems. In J. M. Violanti, D. Paton, & C. Dunning (Eds.), *Posttraumatic Stress Intervention: Challenges, Issues and Perspectives* (pp. 81–96). Springfield, IL: Charles C Thomas.

Hart, P. M., & Wearing, A. J. (1995). Occupational stress and well-being: A systematic approach to research, policy and practice. In P. Cotton (Ed.), *Psychological Health in the Workplace* (pp. 185–216). Carlton: Australian Psychological Society.

Johnston, P., & Paton, D. (2003). Environmental resilience: Psychological empowerment in high-risk professions. In D. Paton, J. M. Violanti, & L. Smith (Eds.), *Promoting Capabilities to Manage Posttraumatic Stress: Perspectives on Resilience* (pp. 136–151). Springfield, IL: Charles C Thomas.

Klein, G. (1996). The effect of acute stressors on decision making. In J. Driskell & E. Salas (Eds.), *Stress and Human Performance.* Hillsdale, NJ: Lawrence Erlbaum.

Klein, G. (1997). Recognition-primed decision making. In C. Zsambok & G. Klein (Eds.), *Naturalistic Decision Making.* Mahwah, NJ: Lawrence Erlbaum.

Lyons, R. F., Mickelson, K. D., Sullivan, M. J. L., & Coyne, J. C. (1998). Coping as a communal process. *Journal of Social and Personal Relationships, 15,* 579–605.

MacLeod, M. D. (2000). The future is always brighter: Temporal orientation and adjustment to trauma. In J. M. Violanti, D. Paton, & C. Dunning (Eds.), *Posttraumatic Stress Intervention: Challenges, Issues and)Perspectives* (pp. 166–186). Springfield, IL: Charles C Thomas.

MacLeod, M. D., & Paton, D. (1999). Police officers and violent crime: Social psychological perspectives on impact and recovery. In J. M. Violanti & D. Paton (Eds.), *Police Trauma: Psychological Aftermath of Civilian Combat* (pp. 25–36). Springfield, IL: Charles C Thomas.

Marks, M. A., Sabella, M. J., Burke, C. S., & Zaccaro, S. J. (2002). The impact of cross-training on team effectiveness. *Journal of Applied Psychology, 87,* 3–13.

Mitchell, M. (1991). The police after Lockerbie: What were the effects? *Police, 23,* 30–31.

Moran, C. (1999). Recruits' prediction of positive reactions in disaster and emergency work. *Disaster Prevention and Management, 8,* 177–183.

Moran, C., & Colless, E. (1995). Positive reactions following emergency and disaster responses. *Disaster Prevention and Management, 4,* 55–61.

Orasanu, J. (1997). Stress and naturalistic decision making: Strengthening the weak links. In R. Flin, E. Salas, M. Strub, & L. Martin (Eds.), *Decision Making under Stress* (pp. 43–66). Aldershot: Ashgate.

Orasanu. J., & Backer, P. (1996). Stress and military performance. In J. Driskell & E. Salas (Eds.), *Stress and Performance* (pp. 89–125). Hillsdale, NJ: Lawrence Erlbaum.

Park, C. L. (1998). Stress-related growth and thriving through coping: The roles of personality and cognitive processes. *Journal of Social Issues, 54,* 267–277.

Paton, D. (1989). Disasters and helpers: Psychological dynamics and implications for counselling. *Counselling Psychology Quarterly, 2,* 303–321.

Paton, D. (1994). Disaster relief work: An assessment of training effectiveness. *Journal of Traumatic Stress, 7,* 275–288.

Paton, D. (1997). *Dealing with Traumatic Incidents in the Workplace* (3rd ed.). Queensland, Australia: Gull Publishing.

Paton, D., Cox, D. E. H., & Andrew, C. (1989). A preliminary investigation into stress in rescue workers. R.G.I.T. *Applied Social Science Report,* No. 1.

Paton, D., & Flin, R. (1999). Disaster stress: An emergency management perspective. *Disaster Prevention and Management, 8,* 261–267.

Paton, D., & Jackson, D. (2002). Developing disaster management capability: An assessment centre approach. *Disaster Prevention and Management, 11,* 115–122.

Paton, D., Johnston, D., & Houghton, B. (1998). Organisational responses to a volcanic eruption. *Disaster Prevention and Management, 7,* 5–13.

Paton, D., Johnston, D., Houghton, B., Flin, R., Ronan, K., & Scott, B. (1999a). Managing natural hazard consequences: Information management and decision making. *Journal of the American Society of Professional Emergency Managers, 6,* 37–48.

Paton, D., Smith, L. M., Ramsay, R., & Akande, D. (1999). A structural re-assessment of the Impact of Event Scale: The influence of occupational and cultural contexts. In R. Gist & B. Lubin (Eds.), *Response to Disaster: Psychosocial, Community and Ecological Approaches* (pp. 83–100). Philadelphia: Taylor & Francis.

Paton, D., & Stephens, C. (1996). Training and support for emergency responders. In D. Paton & J. M. Violanti (Eds.), *Traumatic Stress in Critical Occupations: Recognition, Consequences and Treatment* (pp. 173–205). Springfield, IL: Charles C Thomas.

Paton, D., & Violanti, J. M. (Eds.). (1996). *Traumatic Stress in Critical Occupations: Recognition, Consequences and Treatment.* Springfield, IL: Charles C Thomas.

Paton, D., Violanti, J. M., & Smith, L. M. (2003). *Promoting Capabilities to Manage Posttraumatic Stress: Perspectives on Resilience.* Springfield, IL: Charles C Thomas.

Pollock, C., Paton, D., Smith, L., & Violanti, J. M. (2003). Team resilience. In D. Paton, J. M. Violanti, & L. Smith. (Eds.), *Promoting Capabilities to Manage Posttraumatic Stress: Perspectives on Resilience* (pp. 74–88). Springfield, IL: Charles C Thomas.

Powell, T. C. (1991). Shaken, but alive: Organisational behaviour in the wake of catastrophic events. *Industrial Crisis Quarterly, 5,* 271–291.

Raphael, B. (1986). *When Disaster Strikes.* London: Hutchinson.

Raphael, B., & Middleton, W. (1987). Mental health responses in a decade of disasters: Australia 1974–1983. *Hospital and Community Psychiatry, 38,* 1331–1337.

Salas, E., Fowlkes, J. E., Stout, R. J. Milanovich, D. M., & Prince, C. (1999). Does CRM training improve teamwork skills in the cockpit? Two evaluation studies. *Human Factors, 41,* 326–343.

Salas, E., Prince, C., Baker, D. P., & Shestra, L. (1995). Situation awareness in team performance: Implications for measurement and training. *Human Factors, 37,* 123–136.

Sarter, N. B., & Woods, D. D. (1991). Situation awareness: A critical but ill-defined phenomenon. International Journal of Aviation Psychology, 1, 45-57.

Shakespeare-Finch, J., Paton, D. & Violanti, J. M. (2003). The family: Resilience resource and resilience needs In D. Paton, J. M. Violanti, & L. Smith. (Eds.), Promoting capabilities to manage posttraumatic stress: Perspectives on resilience (pp. 170-185). Springfield, IL: Charles C Thomas.

Shaw, R. (1997). Decision making under stress: Forming effective police commanders. Police Research and Management, Autumn, 51-59.

Solomon, S. D., & Smith, E. S. (1994). Social support and perceived control as moderators of responses to dioxin and flood exposure. In R. J. Ursano, B. G. McCaughey, & C. S. Fullerton (Eds.), *Individual and Community Responses to Trauma and Disaster* (pp. 179–200). Cambridge: Cambridge University Press.

Stewart, E., & Flin, R. (1996). Taking action. *Policing Today,* December, 14–17.

Stout, R. J., Cannon-Bowers, J. A., Salas, E., & Milanovich, D. M. (1999). Planning, shared mental models and coordinated performance: An empirical link is established. *Human Factors, 41,* 61–71.

Taylor, A. J. W., & Frazer, A. G. (1982). The stress of post-disaster body handling and victim identification. *Journal of Human Stress, 8,* 4–12.

Tedeschi, R. G. & Calhoun, L. G. (2003) Routes to posttraumatic growth through cognitive processing. In D. Paton, J. M. Violanti, & L. Smith. (Eds.), *Promoting Capabilities to Manage Posttraumatic Stress: Perspectives on Resilience* (pp. 12–26). Springfield, IL: Charles C Thomas.

Thompson, J. (1993). Psychological impact of body recovery duties. *Journal of the Royal Society of Medicine, 86,* 628–629.

Violanti, J. M., & Paton, D. (Eds.). (1999). *Police Trauma: Psychological Aftermath of Civilian Combat.* Springfield, IL: Charles C Thomas.

Travillian, K. K., Volpe, C. E., Cannon-Bowers, J. A., & Salas, E. (1993). Cross-training highly interdependent teams: Effects of team processes on team performance. In *Proceedings of the Human Factors and Ergonomics Society 37th Annual Meeting* (pp. 1243–1247). Santa Monica, CA: Human Factors and Ergonomics Society.

Vrij, A., van der Steen, J., & Koppelaar, L. (1994). Aggression of police officers as a function of temperature: An experiment with the fire arms training system. *Journal of Community and Applied Psychology, 4,* 365–370.

Williams, T. (1993). Trauma in the workplace. In J. P. Wilson, & B. Raphael (Eds.), *International Handbook of Traumatic Stress Syndromes* (pp. 925–934). New York: Plenum Press.

Chapter 8

INCREASING RESILIENCY THROUGH SHARED SENSEMAKING: BUILDING HARDINESS IN GROUPS

PAUL T. BARTONE

INTRODUCTION

Hardiness is generally regarded as an individual personality style or trait and has been identified in various studies as an important stress-resistance resource *for individuals.* But many of those who are at risk from traumatic stressors work in cohesive groups, usually with some kind of structure and leadership hierarchy. This is true, for example, for firemen, policemen, military personnel, and various other emergency responders (Pollock, Paton, Smith, & Violanti, 2003). Is there some way to take what is known about hardiness as a personal resiliency resource and apply it to groups? Can we reduce the risk of traumatic stress by increasing resiliency or hardiness in some degree for everyone within the work group?

This chapter argues that it is indeed possible to do this and focuses on military groups as an exemplary case-in-point. I begin by describing the nature of stressors encountered by soldiers on modern military operations. Next, I explain the hardiness construct in some detail and summarize recent research showing that hardiness reduces the risk for stress-related psychological injury. I suggest that the essential underlying mechanism in the hardiness–stress resiliency process involves how stressful events get interpreted or "made-sense" of, and that this "sensemaking" process can be influenced by group leaders in various ways. This provides an avenue for applying hardiness concepts toward the goal of reducing risk in high-stress groups. A brief case report from a recent military operation is offered to elucidate how this process might occur. Finally, I provide some recommendations for leader actions aimed at building up hardiness in groups.

THE NATURE OF STRESSORS IN MODERN MILITARY OPERATIONS

Compared with earlier times, military operations in the post-Cold War era are different in a number of ways. Soldiers are going away on more deployments than ever before. This phenomenon is sometimes characterized in military circles as "high operations tempo." The high operations tempo in turn is seen as increasing the stress and strain on military forces, perhaps even contributing to readiness and retention problems (Castro & Adler, 1999). Increased deployments always entail other stressful changes in military units as well, such as an increased number (and intensity) of training exercises, planning sessions, and equipment inspections, all of which increase the pace of operations. The associated problem is that the stressors associated with modern military operations are experienced at a higher frequency and intensity by soldiers who are deploying more often and for longer periods (Bell, Bartone, Bartone, Schumm & Gade, 1997).

The most obvious way to reduce stress associated with a high operations tempo is to lessen the frequency and duration of deployments. While this may be a reasonable policy goal, it is not always possible within mission constraints. The same is true in other occupations and contexts. For example, following the 9/11 terrorist strike on the World Trade Center, fire, police, and other emergency personnel necessarily maintained continuous operations around the clock with the goals of locating possible survivors and restoring essential services to the affected areas. This leads to the question: What factors, at individual and group levels, can be strengthened or reduced in order to facilitate healthy responding to operational stress hazards? In order to answer this question with respect to the military case, it helps to have a more detailed understanding of the nature of the stressors encountered by soldiers on modern military deployments that are stressful for those performing them.

Interviews, observations, and surveys conducted with United States Army soldiers deployed to Croatia and Bosnia from 1993 through 1996 have identified five primary stressor dimensions on modern military operations: (1) isolation, (2) ambiguity, (3) powerlessness, (4) boredom, and (5) danger (Bartone, Adler, & Vaitkus, 1998; Bartone, 2001).

PERSONALITY HARDINESS AND WHY IT IS IMPORTANT

What personal or group elements might protect soldiers from these dimensions of stress? Hardiness, a measure of resiliency in the face of hardship or danger, may be one such protective trait.

Conceptually, hardiness is a personality dimension that develops early in life and is reasonably stable over time, although amenable to change and probably trainable under certain conditions (Kobasa, 1979; Maddi & Kobasa, 1984). Hardy persons have a high sense of life and work *commitment*, a greater feeling of *control*, and are more open to change and *challenges* in life. They tend to interpret stressful and painful experiences as a normal aspect of existence, a part of life that, overall, is interesting and worthwhile. Since 1979, a fairly extensive body of research has accumulated showing that hardiness protects against the ill effects of stress on health and performance. Research studies with a variety of occupational groups have found that hardiness appears to function as a significant moderator or buffer of stress (Contrada, 1989; Kobasa, Maddi & Kahn, 1982; Roth et al., 1989; Wiebe, 1991).

In military groups, hardiness also has been identified as a significant moderator of combat exposure stress in US Gulf War soldiers (Bartone, 1993; Bartone, 1999; Bartone, 2000). Hardiness has appeared as a stress buffer in other military groups as well, including US Army casualty assistance workers (Bartone et al., 1989), peacekeeping soldiers (Bartone, 1996), Israeli soldiers in combat training (Florian, Mikulincer, & Taubman, 1995), Israeli officer candidates (Westman, 1990), and Norwegian Navy cadets (Bartone, Johnsen, Eid, Laberg, & Brun, 2002). Figure 8-1 shows results from a study on hardiness, combat stress, and PTSD symptoms in United States soldiers who fought in the Gulf War (Bartone, 2000).

Figure 8-1 illustrates the typical and rather robust hardiness X stress interaction effect, wherein it is under high-stress conditions that the resiliency effects of hardiness are most apparent. In this study, high-hardy US Army soldiers exposed to combat stress in the Gulf War showed significantly fewer traumatic stress symptoms (as assessed by the Impact of Events Scale; Horowitz, Wilner, & Alvarez, 1979).

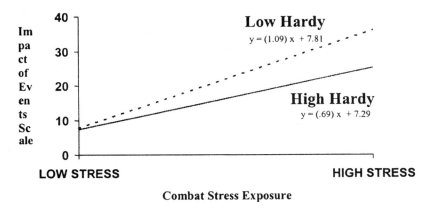

Figure 8-1. Gulf War Combat Stress Exposure (CSE) scores for Low and High Hardy active duty. (Displays Hardy × CSE interaction ($p < 0.0001$) in regression model, $N = 824$ active duty, unstandardized betas used to map regression lines.)

Hardiness – which I construe as a personality style or tendency, reasonably stable over time and across situations – is really not a new concept. It is theoretically grounded in the work of existential philosophers and psychologists like Heidegger (1986), Frankl (1960), and Binswanger (1963) and involves how meaning gets constructed in life (even life that is sometimes painful), and having the courage to live life fully. It is a global concept which affects views of self, others, work, and the physical world (in existentialist terms: *Umwelt*, the "around" world; *Mitwelt*, the "with" or social world; and *Eigenwelt*, the world of the self or me). Without using the term "hardiness," over 30 years ago Maddi (1967) nevertheless outlined the hardy personality type, contrasting it with the nonhardy "existential neurotic." He used the term "ideal identity" to describe the person who lives a vigorous and proactive life, with a strong sense of meaning and purpose, and belief in his own ability to influence things.

Later, Maddi and Kobasa (1984) describe hardiness as a generalized personality style that develops mainly as a function of early life experiences and parent-child interactions. If this is true, then it is something that is basically fixed beyond a certain point and cannot be trained or modified. Or can it? In fact, some research findings as well as theoretical considerations lead me to believe that hardiness levels can be increased to some degree, even in adults. For example, using a structured intervention program, Maddi (1987) successfully increased hardiness levels in corporate managers, and at the same time he found that their physiological responses to stress were tempered and more healthy.

Maddi and colleagues have followed up this work with more refined "hardiness induction" programs that appear to work. In considerations of the question of how to develop hardiness in soldiers and other high-stress work groups, it is important to take a close look at what hardiness is and to consider how it might operate as a stress resiliency factor.

A critical aspect of the hardiness resiliency mechanism likely involves the interpretation or the meaning that people attach to events around them and to their own place in this world of experiences. High-hardy people will typically interpret experience as (1) overall interesting and worthwhile, (2) something they can exert control over, and (3) challenging, presenting opportunities to learn and grow.

It seems probable that in military units, this "meaning-making" process is something that leaders can influence. Military units are by their nature group-oriented and highly interdependent. The typical tasks and missions are group ones. And the hierarchical authority structure puts leaders in a position to exercise substantial control and influence over subordinates. By the policies and priorities they establish, the directives they give, the advice and counsel they offer, the stories they tell, and perhaps most importantly the example they set, leaders may indeed alter the manner in which their subordinates interpret and make sense of their experiences.

CASE STUDY: HOW THE HARDY LEADER INCREASES GROUP HARDINESS ON MODERN MILITARY MISSIONS

Many authors have considered the ways in which group and organizational processes might influence how meaning gets constructed at the individual level. For example, Berger and Luckmann (1966) discuss compellingly how much of what we perceive in our everyday lives is the result of basic social processes, essentially "social constructions" that take on a quality of permanent reality. Consider also Irving Janis' (1982) demonstrated process of "groupthink," in which individuals conform to the dominant perspective of their group, even in the face of disconfirming evidence. Even Gordon Allport (1985), the eminent American personality psychologist, viewed individual meaning as often an essentially social construction. The organizational psychologist Karl Weik (1995) uses the term "sensemaking" to describe the process of (often retrospective) interpretation of events, especially ambiguous ones, by individuals and groups in organizations. It would seem that peers, leaders, and indeed the entire unit or organizational culture can influence how experiences get interpreted.

Two recent studies done with military cadets training to be officers lend some support to the notion that leaders high in hardiness may influence their subordinates to think and behave in more hardy/resilient ways. The first study, with West Point cadets, shows simply that hardiness levels are related significantly to leader performance, as rated by several supervisors.

To measure hardiness, this study used a 15-item scale that included both positively and negatively keyed items, and covered the three hardiness facets of commitment, control, and challenge (Bartone et al., 1989; Bartone, 1995). The short hardiness scale was administered to a single West Point cohort during spring of their senior year (Bartone, 1998), with a response rate of 50% (N = 435). Cronbach's alpha coefficient for the total measure is 0.70 in this sample. In another group of college students (West Point; N = 105), the three-week test-retest reliability coefficient was 0.78. Leader performance was assessed with "Military Development" (MD) grades, which are assigned to cadets at the end of each academic semester at West Point. These grades represent an average of leader performance ratings given by an officer supervisor and the ratings of 2–3 cadet (upperclassmen) supervisors (US Corps of Cadets, 1995). Results of a multiple regression analysis predicting cumulative MD across four years (Multiple R = 0.23, F (8, 1141) = 11.95, p < 0.001) identified as significant predictors hardiness, transformational leadership, College Entrance Examination scores, social judgment, emotional stability (–), extraversion, and traditional values (Table 8-1).

Personality hardiness emerges as the strongest and most consistent predictor of military development grades for these officer cadets. These results indicate that people who are higher in hardiness – a characteristic sense of commitment, control, and challenge – are more effective in positions of leadership in a military organization.[1] In a related study, hardiness was found to be an even stronger predictor of leader performance for female West Point cadets (Bartone & Snook, 1999).

---

[1] Transformational leadership style (Bass, 1998; Burns, 1978) enters the regression model as a significant independent predictor of leader performance. A correlational analysis reveals that transformational leadership is not significantly correlated with hardiness, although transformational leadership is moderately correlated with the hardiness facet of commitment. It is possible that cadets high in personality hardiness are more apt to develop a transformational leadership style, but that this will occur only under certain environmental or organizational conditions.

TABLE 8-1
LEADERSHIP (MD) PREDICTORS, WEST POINT, 4 YEARS TOTAL

Predictor	Beta	t	p <
Hardiness	0.15	5.1	0.00
Transformational leadership	0.11	3.9	0.00
College entrance scores	0.07	2.5	0.01
Social judgment	0.07	2.3	0.02
Emotional stability	−0.07	−2.2	0.03
Extraversion	0.07	2.0	0.04
Traditional values	0.07	2.0	0.04

Multiple regression, backward elimination, mean substitution for missing data
Model: $F_{(8, 1141)} = 11.95$, $p < 0.0001$; Multiple $R = 0.23$; R square $= 0.06$

Findings from a recent study done with Norwegian Navy cadets are even more suggestive of a "hardy leader effect" within the group. One purpose of this study was to identify factors that contributed to the development of cohesion in squad-sized navy officer cadet units undergoing an intense 2-week training exercise. Findings showed that the experience of the stressful exercise itself had a positive effect on team cohesion and that this effect was greater if the groups were already familiar with each other before the exercise (Table 8-2). But we also found that hardiness and small unit leadership influenced cohesion levels in a positive direction and that hardiness and leadership interacted in influencing cohesion (Bartone, Johnsen, Eid, Laberg, & Brun, 2002).

TABLE 8-2
STEPWISE REGRESSION RESULTS, PREDICTING COHESION LEVELS
AFTER A STRESSFUL TRAINING EXERCISE*

Predictor Variable	Beta	t	p <
Rated leadership	0.30	2.4	0.02
Hardiness X leadership	0.29	2.3	0.02

* Hardiness and leadership interact to predict small unit cohesion following a stressful training exercise.
Model: $F_{(2,83)} = 17.4$, $p < 0.001$; Multiple $R = 54$; $R^2 = 0.29$
N = 85 Norwegian Navy officer cadets, 1998

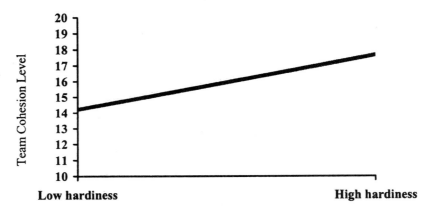

Figure 8-2. Influence of hardiness on T2 Cohesion levels (plotted regression line: $y = B(0.0954) + 14.214$).

Figure 8-2 shows the plotted regression line of hardiness predicting leadership. Group cohesion is significantly higher when hardiness is higher.

In the same study, the combined effects of hardiness and leadership on cohesion levels following stressful exercise were examined. Results showed that the highest scores on team cohesion were observed when unit leadership was perceived as positive and when hardiness levels were also high.

To summarize, the study of Norwegian Navy officer cadets showed mainly that undergoing a stressful training exercise increases small unit cohesion, especially when group members are already familiar with one another. But the study also identified potent effects of leadership at the small unit level on cohesion assessed just after the stressful exercise. This suggests that what leaders do, and how they are perceived by their subordinates, can have a team-building or cohesion-enhancing effect on the unit. An additional finding, that personality hardiness is also associated with higher cohesion levels in the wake of a stressful group experience, further suggests a "sensemaking" mechanism for such leader effects.

The key operative power of hardiness to buffer or transform stressful experiences seems to be related to the particular interpretations of such experiences that are typically made by the hardy person. If a stressful or painful experience can be cognitively framed and made-sense-of within a broader perspective which holds that all of existence is essentially interesting, worthwhile, fun, and a matter of personal choice and provides chances to learn and grow, then the stressful experience can have beneficial psychological effects instead of harmful ones.

In a small group context, leaders are in a unique position to shape how stressful experiences are understood by members of the group. The leader who, through example and discussion, communicates a positive construction or reconstruction of shared stressful experiences may exert an influence on the entire group in the direction of his/her interpretation of experience. Thus, leaders high in hardiness are likely have a greater impact in their groups under high-stress conditions when by their example, as well as through the explanations they may articulate to group members, they encourage an interpretation of stressful events as interesting challenges which they are capable of meeting and, in any event, can learn and benefit from. This process itself, as well as the positive result of the process (a shared understanding of the event as something worthwhile and beneficial), could also be expected to generate an increased sense of shared values, mutual respect, and cohesion. The regression results showing hardiness and leadership interacting to explain post-exercise cohesion levels lend support to this interpretation.

As we have seen, there is some data to support the view that hardy leaders can generate increasingly "hardy" and positive shared interpretations of experience, at least in the context of stressful training exercises. Can this valuable leader influence apply in other circumstances such as mass casualties or disasters, or modern military deployments that entail the kinds of stressors outlined earlier (isolation, ambiguity, powerlessness, boredom, danger)? I believe the answer to this question is yes, although we are still in the early stages of understanding this influence process and the circumstances under which it might operate.

Although more research is certainly needed to understand the mechanisms of group resiliency and sensemaking, we can nevertheless point to a number of actions that leaders may take to build hardiness and resiliency in high-stress work groups:

1. Lead by example; provide subordinates with a model of the hardy approach to life and work. Through actions and words, demonstrate a strong sense of commitment, control, and challenge, and a perspective on stressful circumstances that says stress can be valuable, and always at least provides an opportunity to learn and grow.

2. Facilitate "hardy" group sensemaking of experience in (a) how tasks or missions are planned, discussed, and executed; (b) how mistakes, failures, and casualties are spoken about and interpreted; and (c)

debriefings and "After-Action Reviews," by focusing on events as learning opportunities and making positive constructions of events as well as responses that occurred around the event.

3. Seek out (create if necessary!) meaningful/challenging group tasks, and then capitalize on group accomplishments by providing recognition, awards, and opportunities to reflect on results (e.g., photographs, news accounts, and other tangible mementos).

CONCLUSION

In work groups such as the military, where individuals in groups are regularly exposed to extreme work-related stressors and hazards, leaders are in a unique position to shape how stressful experiences are made sense of, or interpreted and understood by members of the group. The leader who, through example and discussion, communicates a positive construction or reconstruction of shared stressful experiences exerts an influence on the entire group in the direction of his/her interpretation of experience – toward more resilient and hardy sensemaking. This positive effect is likely to be greater, the greater the isolation of the group and the intensity of the stressful situation. For occupational groups that routinely and necessarily are exposed to extreme and sometimes prolonged stressors, including police, fire, emergency, and military personnel, avoiding stressors is usually not an option. They all must work under conditions that place them "in harm's way," exposed to a range of hazards and psychological risks. But the potential for negative stress consequences can be reduced by drawing on the concepts of hardiness theory, particularly constructive sensemaking of stressful experiences, and using these to inform leader actions and group risk management approaches.

REFERENCES

Allport, G. W. (1985). The historical background of social psychology. In G. Lindzey, & E. Aronson (Eds.), *Handbook of Social Psychology* (3rd ed., Vol. 1, pp. 1–46). New York: Random House.

Bartone, P. T. (1996, August). *Stress and hardiness in U.S. peacekeeping soldiers.* Paper presented at the Convention of the American Psychological Association, Toronto, Canada.

Bartone, P. T. (1989). Predictors of stress-related illness in city bus drivers. *Journal of Occupational Medicine, 31,* 657–663.

Bartone, P. T. (1993, June). *Psychosocial predictors of soldier adjustment to combat stress.* Paper presented at the Third European Conference on Traumatic Stress, Bergen, Norway.

Bartone, P. T. (1995, July). *A short hardiness scale.* Paper presented at the Annual Convention of the American Psychological Society, New York.

Bartone, P. T. (1998). Test-retest reliability of a short hardiness scale. Unpublished manuscript, Department of Behavioral Sciences and Leadership, U.S. Military Academy, West Point, New York.

Bartone, P. T. (1999). Hardiness protects against war-related stress in Army reserve forces. *Consulting Psychology Journal, 51,* 72–82.

Bartone, P. T. (2000). Hardiness as a resiliency factor for United States Forces in the Gulf War. In J. M. Violanti, D. Paton, & C. Dunning (Eds.), *Posttraumatic Stress Intervention: Challenges, Issues, and Perspectives* (pp. 115–133). Springfield, IL: Charles C Thomas.

Bartone, P. T. (2001, June). *Psychosocial stressors in future military operations.* Paper presented at the Cantigny Conference Series on Future of Armed Conflict, Wheaton, Illinois.

Bartone, P. T., Adler, A. B. & Vaitkus, M. A. (1998). Dimensions of psychological stress in peacekeeping operations. *Military Medicine, 163,* 587–593.

Bartone, P. T., Johnsen, B. H., Eid, J., Laberg, J. C. & Brun, W. (2002). Factors influencing small unit cohesion in Norwegian Navy Officer cadets. *Military Psychology, 14,* 1–22.

Bartone, P. T., & Snook, S. A. (1999, May). *Cognitive and personality factors predict leader development in U.S. Army cadets.* Paper presented at the 35th International Applied Military Psychology Symposium (IAMPS), Florence, Italy.

Bartone, P. T., Ursano, R. J., Wright. K. W,. & Ingraham, L. H. (1989). The impact of a military air disaster on the health of assistance workers: A prospective study. *Journal of Nervous and Mental Disease, 177,* 317–328.

Bass, B. M. (1998). *Transformational Leadership.* Mahwah, NJ: Lawrence Erlbaum.

Bell, D. B., Bartone, J., Bartone, P. T., Schumm, W. R., & Gade, P. A. (1997). *USAREUR family support during Operation Joint Endeavor: Summary report* (ARI Special Report 34). Alexandria, VA: U. S. Army Research Institute for the Behavioral and Social Sciences. ADA339016.

Berger, P. L., & Luckmann, T. (1966). *The Social Construction of Reality.* Garden City, NY: Doubleday.

Binswanger, L. (1963). *Being in the World: Selected Papers of Ludwig Binswanger.* New York: Basic Books.

Burns, J. M. (1978). *Leadership.* New York: Harper & Row.

Castro, C., & Adler, A. (1999). OPTEMPO: Effects on soldier and unit readiness. *Parameters, 29,* 86–95.

Contrada, R. J. (1989). Type A behavior, personality hardiness, and cardiovascular responses to stress. *Journal of Personality and Social Psychology, 57,* 895–903.

Florian, V., Mikulincer, M., & Taubman, O. (1995). Does hardiness contribute to mental health during a stressful real life situation? The role of appraisal and coping. *Journal of Personality and Social Psychology, 68,* 687–695.

Frankl, V. (1960). *The doctor and the Soul.* New York: Knopf.

Heidegger, M. (1986). *Being and Time.* New York: Harper Collins Publishers.

Horowitz, M., Wilner, N., & Alvarez, W. (1979). Impact of Events Scale: A measure of subjective stress. *Psychosomatic Medicine, 41,* 209–218.

Ingraham, L. H., & Manning, F. J. (1981). Cohesion: Who needs it, what is it and how do we get it to them? *Military Review, 61,* 3–12.

Janis, I. (1982). *Groupthink* (2d ed.). Boston: Houghton Mifflin.

Kirkland, F. R., Bartone, P. T., & Marlowe, D. H. (1993). Commanders' priorities and psychological readiness. *Armed Forces and Society, 19,* 579–598.

Kobasa, S. C. (1979). Stressful life events, personality, and health: An inquiry into hardiness. *Journal of Personality and Social Psychology, 37,* 1–11.

Kobasa, S. C., & Maddi, S. R. (1977). Existential personality theory. In R. Corsini (Ed.), *Existential Personality Theories.* Itasca, IL: Peacock.

Kobasa, S. C., Maddi, S. R., & Kahn, S. (1982). Hardiness and health: A prospective study. *Journal of Personality & Social Psychology, 42,* 168–177.

Maddi, S. R. (1967). The existential neurosis. *Journal of Abnormal Psychology, 72,* 311–325.

Maddi, S. R. (1987). Hardiness training at Illinois Bell Telephone. In J. P. Opatz (Ed.), *Health Promotion Evaluation.* Stephens Point, Wisconsin: National Wellness Institute.

Maddi, S. R., & Kobasa, S. C. (1984). *The Hardy Executive.* Homewood, IL: Dow Jones-Irwin.

Paton, D. (1997). Managing work-related psychological trauma: An organizational psychology of response and recovery. *Australian Psychologist, 32,* 46–55.

Pollock, C., Paton, D., Smith, L., & Violanti, J. (2003). Team Resilience. In D. Paton, J. Violanti, & L. Smith (Eds.), *Promoting Capabilities to Manage Posttraumatic Stress: Perspectives on Resilience.* Springfield, IL: Charles C Thomas.

Roth, D. L., Wiebe, D. J., Fillingim, R. B., & Shay, K. A. (1989). Life events, fitness, hardiness, and health: A simultaneous analysis of proposed stress-resistance effects. *Journal of Personality and Social Psychology, 57,* 136–142.

U.S. Corps of Cadets (1995). *Leadership evaluation and developmental ratings.* (USCC Regulation 623-1). West Point, New York: United States Military Academy.

Weik, K. E. (1995). *Sensemaking in Organizations.* Thousand Oaks, CA: Sage.

Weisaeth, L., & Sund, A. (1982). Psychiatric problems in UNIFIL and the UN-Soldier's stress syndrome. *International Review of Army, Air Force and Navy Medical Service, 55,* 109–116.

Westman, M. (1990). The relationship between stress and performance: The moderating effect of hardiness. *Human Performance, 3,* 141–155.

Wiebe, D. J. (1991). Hardiness and stress moderation: A test of proposed mechanisms. *Journal of Personality and Social Psychology, 60,* 89–99.

Chapter 9

DISASTER RESPONSE: RISK FACTORS IN AN INTERNATIONAL CONTEXT

Douglas Paton, A. J. W. Taylor, and Colleen McFarlane

INTRODUCTION

If disasters, whether of natural or human origin, occur in countries lacking the means to meet the unique needs of survivors and communities, a response from the international community will ensue. Consequently, emergency service, mental health, medical, military, and humanitarian aid personnel are increasingly becoming involved in disaster relief and peacekeeping roles overseas. When involved in this capacity, they operate within a context characterized by, for example, exposure to death, personal danger, unique cultural attitudes and practices, isolation, poverty, political conflict, and instability. Furthermore, they may have to do so for prolonged periods of time. This chapter discusses stress risk factors associated with working in this capacity. It does so by drawing upon the experiences of search and rescue workers, medical and mental health professionals, military peacekeepers, and humanitarian aid workers.

DEPLOYMENT

Deployment for international relief work influences stress risk in several ways. Some relate to its more complex nature; others can be attributed to delays and to its duration. When disaster occurs in geographically remote locations, the inevitable delays in deployment represent a significant stress risk factor (Paton, 1994; Paton, Cox, & Andrew, 1989). This problem may be compounded by political inactivity and procrastination as governments evaluate their ability to deal with the crisis and the political costs of calling in outside aid (Comfort, 1999; Paton, 1994; Paton et al., 1989). Using the time afforded by such delays to collect information from the disaster location helps to develop realistic appreciation of the demands likely to be encountered and to adapt plans accordingly that can mitigate stress risk (Paton, 1994).

For mental health workers, deployment will be delayed until summoned by a responsible authority. Contacting colleagues operating in the locality and planning how to integrate their experience with ongoing intervention can mitigate stress risk. They should ensure that their professional credentials will be recognized by the appropriate authority in the host country. They should also address issues relating to the continuity of their practice during their absence and check that the terms of their professional insurance cover them for disaster work overseas. By attending to issues pertaining to their personal relationships, they can minimize the strain that might arise in that quarter.

For some groups, the period of deployment can be measured in weeks (e.g., search and rescue, crisis medical teams). For others, such as aid workers, it can span several months and sometimes years. There are critical points in each phase of overseas work: prior to departure; during the first overseas assignment; and at the time of arrival in the country of assignment, termination of the assignment, and return home (Cardozo & Salama, 2002; McFarlane, 2003b; Shakespeare-Finch, Paton & Violanti, 2003; Sheik et al., 2000). In a peacekeeper sample, McDonald et al. (1996) found that the most anxious times were before and after deployment, with the former colored by anticipatory anxiety and the latter by family and resettlement problems. Homecoming has also been identified as a risk period for adjustment difficulties (Eriksson et al., 2001; McFarlane, 2003b; Sangster, 1996; Shakespeare-Finch et al., 2003), and organizational support upon return home has been noticeably lacking (Danieli, 2002; Macnair, 1995; McCall & Salama, 1999; Moresky et al., 2001; Shakespeare-Finch et al., 2003).

For search and rescue and crisis medical teams deployed during the initial response phase, the sheer scale and urgency of the needs encountered result in their working long days, increasing the risk of physical and mental exhaustion. Rest breaks are essential and should be used constructively (e.g., providing feedback, planning future activities)

(Paton & Stephens, 1996). Breaks can also be used to monitor personnel and make decisions about whether workers should be withdrawn, either temporarily or permanently, if their reactions suggest they risk developing more serious problems or when it is considered that they represent a risk to other team members.

Mental health professionals must also guard against fatigue by doing what they can to moderate the demands made of them. Physical and emotional exhaustion soon leads to burnout, and it underscores the need for health professionals to keep an eye on themselves and their colleagues to prevent it from occurring.

CONTRASTING CONDITIONS

Disaster relief and aid work exposes personnel to environments whose characteristics and demands stand in sharp contrast to those they are accustomed to in their home country. Stress risk is strongly linked to the ease and the degree to which atypical factors can be assimilated into the operational schemata that facilitate comprehension of experiences, generate expectations regarding, roles, tasks, events, environmental characteristics, and the outcomes of the work (Barron, 1999; Paton, 1994).

Expectations regarding the applicability of routine command and control mechanisms can be thwarted by the scale of disruption and the need to deal with atypical, emergent, and often escalating demands (Paton, 1989; Paton, 1994; Paton & Flin, 1999). Effective mitigation requires a shift from autocratic, directive management to a more cooperative and participative style. Similarly, the command expectations of military peacekeepers will be inconsistent with those of large amorphous and remote multinational organizations such as the United Nations. The need to adapt to new organizational or international coordination mechanisms can constitute a stress risk factor.

In their daily work, psychologists respond to the needs of people and groups referred to them in an orderly manner for advice, treatment, and support. But unless they practice predominantly with immigrants and refugees, they rarely attend to the community and cultural concerns they encounter in overseas contexts. These dimensions of human behavior lie beyond the boundaries of conventional training. Similarly, given the rarity of disasters, few health professionals are involved full-time on disaster and emergency work (International Red Cross and Red Crescent Society, 1998).

Risk is influenced by inconsistencies between workers' role expectations and their perception within the host culture (McFarlane, 2003a; Paton & Purvis, 1995). Inexperienced aid workers may wish to be seen by locals as altruistic and helpful, but they can become targets for anger and retribution if, for example, locals perceive their help as inappropriate or inconsistent with their beliefs. It can also extend to having to deal with local attitudes to victims, standards of care, care practices, and grieving rituals and practices (McFarlane, 2003b; Paton & Purvis, 1995). This confrontation of their value system may come at a time when their professional confidence to deal with the situation is most needed (Barron, 1999).

Mental health professionals must contend with other contrasts. For example, they work from temporary facilities where their ability to offer psychological safety and confidentiality is dictated by circumstances beyond their control. They might even have to find such safe havens themselves and adopt outreach methods of approaching survivors who gather of their own accord. When acquiring information, they may need to adopt more of an inquisitorial style than they normally practice and be less reliant on the conventional therapeutic hour for the duration of sessions. Once satisfied as to the physical health of the survivors, psychologists will adopt the triage system in decision making, differentiating between those needing maximum, medium, and minimum help. Contrasts with their routine practice also will be marked by having to make immediate decisions regarding short-term psychological help, while being aware that the initial reactions they see might be unreliable indicators of future chronicity. For purposes of accountability and to prevent their own cognitive overload, they will keep such rudimentary records as circumstances allow and look forward to having a designated supervisor review their performance. Over time, as circumstances allow, the psychologist can resume a more conventional style of practice in familiar settings.

Initially, psychologists may be able to do little more than give factual information about the typical symptoms and signs of traumatic stress (using appropriate language and terminology). They may help reunite survivors with supporting family members and friends and make appropriate referrals to other agencies. Attending to family and sociocultural needs involves uniting survivors with a network of people on whom they can rely for support as they work through their difficulties. Here the clinician cannot be so well informed as to know the variety of relationships that might arise for every person, in every family, in every community, in every culture (Taylor, 2001).

OUTCOMES OF THE RELIEF EFFORT

Relief workers frequently find themselves faced with environmental and organizational factors that result in the outcomes or effectiveness of their endeavors falling short of their expectations. While risk, in this context, can be partially attributed to the scale of loss encountered, it is the tendency to internalize perceived failure to perform at expected levels rather than to attribute it to situational constraints on performance (MacLeod & Paton, 1999) that lies at the source of this problem. Relief workers must acknowledge that atypical external factors can undermine performance effectiveness. Training and review processes should ensure that personnel do not attribute a perceived lessening in effectiveness to inadequacy on their part. Of particular importance is the fact that some of these problems can be attributed to the actions of the relief agency.

Limited organizational preparedness contributes to uncertainty and low role clarity. This, in turn, elevates anticipatory anxiety in international staff prior to departure (McFarlane, 2003a). Conflict with the aid organization (or staff members therein), role ambiguity, the remoteness of the Western office to the in-country office, and the functional capacity of the NGO all increase the risk that unconstructive relationships may impact perceptions of organizational support. Communication difficulties across the geographical divide of field and national offices may be an important mediator in these matters (McFarlane, 2003a; Paton & Purvis, 1995).

Feelings of anger and annoyance and distancing themselves from the aid organization are common reactions when aid workers are disappointed by a lack of support or when they are directed to perform tasks that serve agency imperatives rather than humanitarian goals (McFarlane, 2003a; Paton & Purvis, 1995). This is particularly evident when staff are faced with acute stressors, or when direct requests for assistance are met with unconstructive responses. Distancing between the two parties can reduce responsiveness by one or more parties and compromise more pressing matters such as security.

The onus is on agencies to understand the link between the operating context and the tasks their staff will perform. The imposition of decisions by agencies removed physically and psychologically from the reality of field work compounds the stress risk of relief personnel (Paton & Purvis, 1995). Authority should be devolved to facilitate decision making by those in the field, with the agency acting to support those decisions.

Decisions about what to provide may not be based on an assessment of the actual needs of the affected communities (Comfort, 1999; Paton & Purvis, 1995), and the ensuing community resentment is directed at the relief workers. This reinforces the need to promote realistic expectations with respect to the outcomes of helping activities and to promote the acknowledgment that this reflects situational constraints rather than personal inadequacies.

ROLE STRESS

Role and task conflict and ambiguity are prominent risk factors. They can arise from confronting situations that make atypical demands on competencies or that call the assumptions and beliefs that underpin routine performance into question. It can also be attributed to the need to work with representatives of agencies performing similar or complementary roles and with local professionals and volunteers.

For peacekeepers, a prominent source of role conflict can accompany competing pressures to maintain neutrality while simultaneously remaining ready to intervene forcefully as they reconcile their task as *peacekeepers* with preparing the ground for the *peacemakers*. The term "constabulary ethic" (Moskos, 1975) encapsulates the role stress associated with a shift from the action orientation of peacekeeping to low intensity activities more akin to the role normally performed by the police (Segal, Furukawa, & Lindh, 1990; Segal, Harris, Rothberg, & Marlowe, 1984).

Emergency, health, and welfare professionals from different agencies must act to minimize the risk of professional differences rooted in domestic politics to interfere with the service provided for survivors. Representatives of a particular social service, hospital group, or religious foundation, all of whom may be providing similar services, must not claim exclusive rights of access to disaster casualties. They must also guard against being over-protective of their "professional territory" or squabbling with well-trained and duly appointed volunteers from the local community. While the opportunity to build cross-cultural understanding can make this a beneficial experience if accompanied by a need to reconcile cultural differences in, for example, care practices and attitudes, the risk of negative outcomes is heightened (Paton & Purvis, 1995).

Attempts to project an organizational image can complicate this situation. (Comfort, 1999). Irrespective of the needs of survivors, the organizational response may be driven as much by its underlying philosophy (e.g., as a development agency or religious group) as by its altruistic concerns. This duality can create considerable ambiguity of purpose in the eyes of the representatives of relief agencies and the local community alike.

Role conflict can be fueled by aspects of the political climate within the host country. Humanitarian staff may experience role conflict between their professional goals and those of beneficiaries; local and international governments, particularly when their role is rebuilding peace and security, may work in antithesis to governments that are corrupt, factional, self-interested or dictatorial (McFarlane, 2003a).

Mitigating this problem is difficult. Advance knowledge of the complexities of working in a context characterized by the competing needs and goals of other national and international helping organizations may help defuse problems that result from jealousy or rivalry during the response phase. Agency representatives could liaise to coordinate the operational response to complex disasters. Any mechanism intended to fulfill this function will have to reconcile the differences in attitudes, philosophies, training, and operating techniques that differentiate the teams (Comfort, 1999).

Role stress from the simultaneous activation of helper and victim stereotypes (Short, 1979) can affect aid workers' ability to express emotional care needs in the face of overwhelming demands to give (Blacque-Belair, 2002; Lange, Frankenfield, & Frame, 1994; Sharp et al., 1995). Barron (1999) also noted that "worker-victims typically do not feel entitled to attend to or have others attend to their own needs. Denying their own needs can become second nature or may even have drawn them to relief work in the first place" (p. 156). It can leave the aid worker feeling emotionally isolated. Education about vulnerability and "permission" to be vulnerable needs to be incorporated into every stage of employment. Aid workers may also be reluctant to follow preventive measures for their own health if these measures are not available to the local population (Sharp et al., 1995; Blacque-Belair, 2002).

INFLUENCES ON PHYSICAL AND PSYCHOLOGICAL WELL-BEING

Exposure to threatening circumstances, intentional violence (Sheik et al., 2000), infectious disease (Paton & Purvis, 1995; Peytremann, Baduraux, O'Donovan, & Loutan, 2001), and accidents (Hurlburt, 2002; Schouten & Borgdorff, 1995) represent significant causes of injury, illness, and death in international relief personnel. Search and rescue workers must operate in physically dangerous environments (e.g., buildings damaged by earthquake or explosion). Medical workers face constant exposure to disease and often find themselves working in unsterile conditions. Aid workers face threats of violence (bombings, shootings, assaults, kidnappings, rape, and accidents) that increase risk of posttraumatic stress disorder (PTSD) (Ozer, Best, Lipsey, & Weiss, 2003). Concerns about the personal safety of oneself, one's colleagues, and one's family and friends are common (Eriksson et al., 2001). The neutrality and impartiality conferred onto humanitarians are no longer protective in the chaos of contemporary wars where a lack of legal and military protection for humanitarian staff exacerbates the problem of violence (Smith, 2002). Eriksson (1997) found that a high frequency of exposure to severe occurrences increased the risk of high levels of distress upon return home. Nor does this risk only emanate from external sources; relief workers themselves can play an active role in this process.

Risk-taking behavior (e.g., venturing out into lines of fire for pizza) is prevalent among humanitarian staff (Smith, 2002). Risk addiction associated with long-term exposure to threatening circumstances (Paton, Violanti, & Schmuckler, 1999) can increase the likelihood of relief workers deliberately putting themselves, and sometimes others, into dangerous situations. Sheik et al. (2000) reported that workers who were parents were significantly less likely to die from unintentional violence (accidents), implying that individuals without such responsibilities are more likely to engage in risk-taking behaviors. In addition, host countries often lack infrastructure and regulation, and prevailing norms about risk-taking behavior may differ (McFarlane, 2003b).

Given the context within which relief work takes place, it is not surprising that personnel risk developing significant mental health problems. Eriksson et al. (2001) found that 10% of their sample of returned American relief workers had developed PTSD after 3 years at home, a rate comparable to levels of distress among humanitarian peacekeepers (Weerts et al., 2002). Such outcomes have been linked to prolonged deployment, as well as problems with accommodation, finances, safety, job security, and family dislocation (Ahmad, 2002; Holtz, Salama, Lopes Cardozo, & Gotway, 2002). Encounters with death and loss on a large scale, demands that substantially exceed resource availability, inappropriate management practices, substantive changes in responsibility, constantly having to make difficult decisions, and the political context have been linked to traumatic stress reactions in search and rescue personnel (Paton et al., 1989; Paton, 1994).

The UN has identified three broad types of psychological strain that peacekeepers might experience (United Nations, 1995, Pt. 2). The first concerns typical occupational stressors, discomforts, and deprivations associated with active service assignments in foreign cultures and climates, the reactions to which vary according to a complex of factors involving personal vulnerability, group cohesion, family situations and support, and routine counter-measures for self-management. The second concerns the cumulative effect of occupational strain that, if prolonged, may lead beyond distress to exhaustion and burn-out. The third is attributed to the direct and indirect experience of extraordinary life-threatening or horrific events.

Shigemura and Nomura (2002) reiterate the lack of attention given to the mental health problems of peacekeepers. They refer to the "peacekeeper's stress syndrome" associated with reactions to confronting violence and atrocities to which the peacekeeper could not respond – reactions such as rage, delusion, frustration, feelings of impotence, and helplessness. Bartone, Adler, and Vaitkus (1998) identify isolation, ambiguity, powerlessness, boredom, and threat/danger as the major dimensions of psychological stress. McDonald et al. (1996) describe remaining neutral in the face of strong provocation, frustration from witnessing atrocities and being unable to intervene, being unfamiliar with handling civilian women and children as casualties, the retrieval and disposal of human remains, and the distribution of food to the hungry as significant stressors. While they found that only 3% of peacekeepers needed clinical referral, at greatest risk were the inexperienced, and younger and immature personnel from dysfunctional family backgrounds.

SUPPORT AND TEAM RELATIONS

The interpersonal environment can present its own risk factors. Idiosyncratic habits and disagreements can contribute to a breakdown in team relationships, undermine the quality of the social support available to team members, reduce levels of trust, and compromise security (Paton et al., 1989; Paton & Purvis, 1995; Smith, 2002). Smith (2002) also noted that stressed aid workers tend to form unwise relationships and are more likely to experience conflict with colleagues. Staff conflict disrupts programs.

Social, cultural, and geographical isolation are inherent aspects of the overseas experience and represent significant risk factor for stress and deteriorated well-being. Isolation reduces opportunities for social support, a factor commonly associated with the amelioration of traumatic stress (Davidson, Hughes, Blazer, & George, 1991; Flannery, 1990). Increasing access to electronic communication technology and facilitating the integration of international staff and local people can ameliorate feelings of loneliness and isolation (Hullett & Witte, 2001). This task, however, may not always be straightforward.

The stress associated with isolation is compounded by placement in "high distance" cultures (where humanitarians usually work). This kind of isolation has been associated with lower levels of cultural adaptation and job failure in other groups such as international students and multinational business personnel (Hullett & Witte, 2001; van Oudenhoven, van der Zee, & van Kooten, 2001). These authors recommend cultural training methods to improve cultural empathy, interpersonal problem-solving techniques, and reinforcement of self-efficacious behaviors.

FAMILY AND SIGNIFICANT OTHERS

Relations with significant others at home (spouse, children, elderly parents) can be affected by distance and difficulties of attending to their concerns (Danieli, 2002; Hurlburt, 2002; McFarlane, 2003a; Shakespeare-Finch et al., 2003). Similarly, those at home may have difficulties understanding what the aid worker is going through. Adequate compassion leave for travel (Hurlburt, 2002) and involvement of family members in predeparture training (van Oudenhoven et al., 2001) and on-going organizational activities (Shakespeare-Finch et al., 2003) are recommended.

Family members experience their partners' involvement in unique ways. Specific attention should be directed to them, particularly in regard to the return period. As the period of deployment increases, so too does the level of stress risk associated with the period of return and reintegration (Shakespeare-Finch et al., 2003). This increase in stress risk can be particularly problematic when a team member is seriously injured or killed, and the specific needs that arise under these circumstances should be accommodated when planning for family support needs.

THE POLITICAL ENVIRONMENT

Political expediency exercises a strong influence on the nature, quality, and extent of disaster readiness. Where political will in this regard has been lacking, factors such as inadequate warnings, poor building standards, limited capacity for social and economic continuity, and political instability will add to the complexity of the environment within which relief workers operate (Grigorian, 1992; Paton, 1994; Paton, et al., 1989). In addition to its direct influence on stress risk, the level of infrastructure loss and inadequate systems for assessing needs and distributing resources affects stress risk by influencing both relief workers' perceptions of the effectiveness of their work and the degree of conflict with local community members. Similarly, the redirection of aid to meet political goals may create resentment, exacerbate (pre-existing) political instability, and reduce the coherence of the national response (Harrell-Bond, 1986).

Political Relations Within and Between Countries

Risk from political sources can arise from within donor countries. From the outset, the existence and deployment of peacekeepers have been contentious. Political scientists have questioned the legitimacy of peacekeepers mandates (Bertram, 1995), and pacifists have lobbied politicians and strategists to resolve issues through diplomatic rather than military means (Suter, 1995). Pragmatists have sought clarification of the criteria for determining the contentious locations at which peacekeepers would be deployed, the priority of issues they would address there, the selection of countries supplying the personnel, the size and ethnic mix of the contingents, the duration of deployments, the additional training and support the peacekeepers should receive, the logistics and finance to sustain their operations, the multinational and multilinguistic chains of command, and how their efforts would be evaluated. Finally, peacekeepers have had to contend with the duplicity of politicians whose actual ideological commitment and self-interest are often at variance with that which they declare. Thus the socio-political environment within donor countries can constitute a risk factor through, for example, its influence on attitudes to peacekeeping and peacekeepers.

Agreement to accept help from outside countries can lead to political loss of face, increase threats of internal dissent, reduce the degree of control a government perceives itself as having over its own affairs, and create obligations to other political systems (Raphael, 1986). Even though these problems may be subdued during the disaster, they become significant during the recovery and reconstruction phases and thus represent a prominent source of risk factors for aid workers (Paton & Purvis, 1995).

The quality of political relations between affected and donor countries constitutes a risk factor. Where the quality of relations is poor, governmental procrastination and tardiness about allowing non-national relief agencies into affected areas is more likely. Delays from this quarter increase the complexity of the operating environment. Poor intergovernmental relations also increase the likelihood that relief workers will find themselves interacting with ill-prepared and unsympathetic bureaucracies.

Bureaucracy and Red Tape

The tendency of bureaucratic systems to persist with established procedural rules even when dealing with the different and more urgent demands of a disaster adds complexity to the operating environment as governments strengthen their attempts to maintain control over a situation that they perceive as politically threatening (Comfort, 1999; Paton & Purvis, 1995). This complexity can be further compounded by efforts of the host government to protect itself from criticism and by conflicts regarding internal responsibility for various aspects of the relief effort. The amount of "red tape" that relief workers encounter creates further delays. For instance, they may have to go through official channels to get permission to travel to different sites, experience inadequate national coordination of the relief effort, and suffer poor organization. While their mitigation is well beyond the remit of any relief organization, advising relief workers of these stressors can minimize the psychological consequences. In particular, it is important that workers do not internalize performance constraints emanating from this quarter (Paton & Stephens, 1996).

SELECTION AND TRAINING

The selection and training of disaster relief workers, peacekeepers, and aid workers are issues that have not received the attention they deserve (Moresky et al., 2001; Macnair, 1995; Paton, 1994; Simmonds, Gilbert-Miguet, Siem, Carballo, & Zeric, 1998). Selection decisions have often been based primarily on ensuring that personnel with the functional expertise to meet the (perceived) needs of survivors or local populations are deployed. However, disaster relief agencies have not always been particularly astute in understanding these needs, making inappropriate selection decisions as a consequence (Paton & Purvis, 1995). Differentiating personnel in regard to their prior experience is also important.

Cardozo and Salama (2002) note that "a careful match should be made between the assignment and the level of experience so that inexperienced personnel are not deployed to the most stressful situations" (p. 253). They recommended the use of a formal mentoring system to support newcomers to fieldwork. Peer briefings are likely to assist orientation but must balance alarming information with support mechanisms and procedures (Cardozo & Salama, 2002). The potential for idiosyncratic habits, beliefs, and attitudes to fuel interpersonal tensions and undermine team morale and social support (Paton & Purvis, 1995; Paton et al., 1989) suggests that team member compatibility should receive greater attention within the selection process. The need to eliminate latent "disaster junkies" through selection procedure is also indicated.

Selection decisions based on functional competencies may provide little preparation for the complex social, political, and cultural demands that relief workers will encounter or for psychological issues. For example, military personnel, trained to fight either to defend themselves or to advance the territorial ambitions of their governments, do not necessarily have the required interpersonal skills for establishing ground rules for dialogue between bitter opponents for whom truce was often a brief interlude in an historical saga of mutual combat. Nor are they likely to have training in conflict resolution, mediation, and moral persuasion, or expertise in community restoration in a context of complex cultural and political tensions.

In general, training in stress management, conflict resolution, handling the media, working cross-culturally, and team building should be implicit components of aid worker training (Macnair, 1995; McCall & Salama, 1999; Paton, 1994; Paton & Jackson, 2002). These skills promote individual and team stress resilience and enhance performance capability. Team leaders should also receive training in recognizing potential problems and in managing them before they reach serious proportions.

Relief workers and peacekeepers do not necessarily need to be fluent in foreign languages or sensitive to the different religious beliefs and customs of the cultural groups to which they are assigned. Training must emphasize cross-cultural issues (Doherty 1999; Marsalla 1979; Taylor, 2001). Providing insights into cultural diversity and its possible implications for aid work (e.g., how cultural characteristics affect survivor behavior), as well as into how members of the host country construe mental health and psychological problems, should thus be afforded a prominent place in preparatory programs. The development of an understanding of the needs of children and the elderly (Lafond, 1990) and the classification of disasters and disaster casualties (Taylor, 1999) represent areas worthy of inclusion into training programs.

The National Voluntary Organizations Active in Disasters (NVOAD) (Young, 2001), the National Organization for Victims Assistance (NOVA), the American Red Cross (ARC), the Critical Incident Stress Management Association, and the Green Cross have developed training curricula for disaster mental health professionals. The training that they advocate includes the following:

- Focusing on the clinical signs and symptoms of acute and chronic trauma while being aware of those of other psychiatric disorders

- Differentiating between reactions attributable more to recent trauma than either to unresolved psychiatric disorder or to normal grief
- Indicating the kinds of support that casualties might require at different stages of disaster recovery and making clear where it should be provided
- Acknowledging the spiritual components of behavior
- Outlining procedures by which casualties might be induced to convert their raw sensations into manageable memories
- Ensuring that helpers are sufficiently self-disciplined and responsive to organizational demands to work as required without embarrassment, stress, and fatigue

Not just individuals and teams benefit from training. Clinicians have suggested that there is a culture of denial among some aid organizations as well as a legitimate lack of organizational capacity to cope with the psychosocial challenges that their staff face (Ager, Flapper, van Pietersom, & Simon, 2002). The development of organizational policies and practices designed to safeguard the well-being of personnel and facilitate their effective performance are indicated (Cardozo & Salama, 2002; Paton & Purvis, 1995).

CONCLUSIONS

When disaster occurs in countries ill-prepared for it, the relief aid supplied by the international community is vital to the process of regaining stability for survivors and their communities. Generally, relief workers can adapt to the acute and chronic stressors of their work. Articulating the unique set of demands that relief workers experience provides a framework for developing selection, training, in-field support, reintegration, and organizational practices that facilitate stress resilience. It is vital that the systems developed to manage relief workers are designed to facilitate the performance and well-being of those in the field rather than organizational imperatives. The geographical and cultural distances that characterize this work should also be accommodated within the design and management of support strategies. Moreover, clinical and research programs must accommodate the specific cultural factors of each country in order to be effective. It is imperative to advance *timely, effective, appropriate,* and *coordinated* academic and clinical activities in order to protect the well-being of all disaster relief and humanitarian staff.

REFERENCES

Ager, A., Flapper, E., van Pietersom, T., & Simon, W. (2002). Supporting and equipping national and international humanitarian non-governmental organizations and their workers. In Y. Danieli (Ed.), *Sharing the Front Line and the Back Hills: Peacekeepers, Humanitarian Aid Workers and the Media in the Midst of Crisis* (pp. 194–200). Amityville, NY: Baywood.

Ahmad, M. M. (2002). Who cares? The personal and professional problems of NGO fieldworkers in Bangladesh. *Development in Practice, 12*(2), 177–191

Barron, R. A. (1999). Psychological trauma and relief workers. In J. Leaning, S. M. Briggs, & L. C. Chen (Eds.), *Humanitarian Crises: The Medical and Public Health Response* (pp. 143–175). Cambridge, MA: Harvard University Press.

Bartone, P. T., Adler, A. B. & Vaitkus, A. B. (1998). Dimensions of psychological stress in peacekeeping operations. *Military Medicine, 163,* 587–593.

Bertram, E. (1995). Reinventing governments – the promises and perils of United Nations peace building. *Journal of Conflict Resolution, 39*(3), 387–418.

Birenbaum, R. (1994). Peacekeeping stress prompts new approaches to mental health. *Canadian Medical Association Journal, 151*(10), 1484–1489.

Blacque-Belair, M. (2002). Being knowledgeable can help enormously. In Y. Danieli (Ed.), *Sharing the Front Line and the Back Hills: Peacekeepers, Humanitarian Aid Workers and the Media in the Midst of Crisis* (pp. 201–202). Amityville, NY: Baywood.

Cardozo, B. L., & Salama, P. (2002). Mental health of humanitarian aid workers in complex emergencies. In Y. Danieli (Ed.), *Sharing the Front Line and the Back Hills: Peacekeepers, Humanitarian Aid Workers and the Media in the Midst of Crisis* (pp. 242–257). Amityville, NY: Baywood.

Comfort, L. K. (1999). *Shared Risk: Complex Systems in Seismic Response.* Amsterdam: Pergamon.

Danieli, Y. (Ed.). (2002). *Sharing the Front Line and the Back Hills: International Protectors and Providers: Peacekeepers, Humanitarian Aid Workers and the Media in the Midst of Crisis.* Amityville, NY: Baywood.

Davidson, J. R. T., Hughes, D., Blazer, D. G., & George, L. K. (1991). Post-traumatic stress disorder in the community: An epidemiological study. *Psychological Medicine, 21,* 713–721.

Doherty, G. W. (1999). Cross-cultural counseling in disaster settings. *Australasian Journal of Disaster and Trauma Studies, 2.* Retrieved May 13, 2000, from http://www.massey.ac.nz/~trauma/issues/1999-2/doherty.htm

Eriksson, C. B. (1997). Traumatic exposure and reentry symptomatology in international relief and development personnel. *Dissertation Abstracts International, 58,* 04B.

Eriksson, C. B., Vande Kemp, H., Gorusch, R., Hoke, S., & Foy, D. W. (2001). Trauma exposure and PTSD symptoms in international relief and development personnel. *Journal of Traumatic Stress, 14*(1), 205–212.

Flannery, R. B. (1990). Social support and psychological trauma: A methodological review. *Journal of Traumatic Stress, 3,* 593–611.

Grigorian, H. M. (1992). The Armenian earthquake. In L. S. Austin (Ed.), *Responding to Disaster* (pp. 157–168). Washington, DC: American Psychiatric Press.

Harrell-Bond, B. E. (1986). *Imposing Aid: Emergency Assistance and Refugees.* Oxford: Oxford University Press.

Holtz, T. H., Salama, P., Lopes Cardozo, B., & Gotway, C. A. (2002). Mental health status of human rights workers, Kosovo, June 2000. *Journal of Traumatic Stress, 15*(5), 389–395.

Hullett, C. R., & Witte, K. (2001). Predicting intercultural adaptation and isolation: Using the extended parallel process model to test anxiety/uncertainty management theory. *International Journal of Intercultural Relations, 25,* 125–139.

Hurlburt, K. (2002). Precious lives honored to serve. In Y. Danieli (Ed.), *Sharing the Front Line and the Back Hills: Peacekeepers, Humanitarian Aid Workers and the Media in the Midst of Crisis* (pp. 161–169). Amityville, NY: Baywood.

International Federation of Red Cross and Red Crescent Societies. (1998). *World Disasters Report.* Oxford: Oxford University Press.

Lafond, R. (1990). *Personal Services: Psychosocial Planning for Disasters.* Ottawa: Minister of Supply and Services.

Lange, W. R., Frankenfield, D. L., & Frame, J. D. (1994). Morbidity among refugee relief workers. *Journal of Travel Medicine, 1*(2), 111–112.

MacDonald, C., Chamberlain, K., Long, N., & Mirfin, K. (1996). *Psychological Effects of Peacekeeping Deployments on Military Personnel.* Palmerston North, NZ: Massey University.

MacLeod, M. D., & Paton, D. (1999). Police officers and violent crime: Social psychological perspectives on impact and recovery. In J. M. Violanti, & D. Paton (Eds.), *Police Trauma: Psychological Aftermath of Civilian Combat* (pp. 25–36). Springfield, IL: Charles C Thomas.

Macnair, R. (1995). *Room for improvement: The management and support of relief and development workers* (Relief and Rehabilitation Network No. Network Paper 10). London: Overseas Development Institute.

Marsalla, A. J. (1979). Cross-cultural studies of mental disorders. In A. J. Marsalla, R. J. Sharp, & T. J. Ciborowski (Eds.), *Perspectives on Cross-cultural Psychology* (Ch 11). New York: Academic Press.

McCall, M., & Salama, P. (1999). Selection, training, and support of relief workers: An occupational health issue. *British Medical Journal, 318,* 113–116.

McFarlane, C. (2003a). [Psychological responses of humanitarian aid personnel]. Unpublished raw data.

McFarlane, C. (2003b). *The balance of trauma, stress and resilience by international aid workers: A longitudinal qualitative investigation.* Paper presented at the 10th Annual Conference of The Australasian Society for Traumatic Stress Studies, Hobart, Australia.

Moresky, R. T., Eliades, M. J., Bhirmani, M. A., Bunney, E. B., & VanRooyen, M. J. (2001). Preparing international relief workers for health care in the field: An evaluation of organizational practices *Prehospital and Disaster Medicine, 16*(4), 257–262.

Moskos, C. C. (1975). UN peacekeepers: The constabulary ethic and military professionalism. *Armed Forces & Society, 1*(4), 388–401.

Ozer, E. J., Best, S. R., Lipsey, T. L., & Weiss, D. S. (2003). Predictors of posttraumatic stress disorder and symptoms in adults: A meta-analysis. *Psychological Bulletin, 129*(1), 52–73.

Paton, D. (1989). Disasters and helpers: Psychological dynamics and implications for counselling. *Counselling Psychology Quarterly, 2,* 303–321.

Paton, D. (1994). Disaster relief work: An assessment of training effectiveness. *Journal of Traumatic Stress, 7,* 275–288.

Paton, D., Cox, D., & Andrew, C. (1989). *A preliminary investigation into posttraumatic stress in rescue workers.* RGIT Social Science Research Report, 1.

Paton, D., & Flin, R. (1999). Disaster stress: An emergency management perspective. *Disaster Prevention and Management, 8,* 261–267.

Paton, D., & Jackson, D. (2002). Developing disaster management capability: An assessment centre approach. *Disaster Prevention and Management, 11,* 115–122.

Paton, D., & Purvis, C. (1995). Nursing in the aftermath of disaster: Orphanage relief work in Romania. *Disaster Prevention and Management, 4,* 45–54.

Paton, D., & Stephens, C. (1996). Training and support for emergency responders. In D. Paton, & J. M. Violanti (Eds.), *Traumatic Stress in Critical Occupations: Recognition, Consequences and Treatment* (pp. 173–205). Springfield, IL: Charles C Thomas.

Paton, D., Violanti, J. & Schmuckler, E. (1999). Chronic exposure to risk and trauma: Addiction and separation issues in police officers. In J. M. Violanti, & D. Paton (Eds.), *Police Trauma: Psychological Aftermath of Civilian Combat.* Springfield, IL: Charles C Thomas.

Peytremann, I., Baduraux, M., O'Donovan, S., & Loutan, L. (2001). Medical evacuations and fatalities of United Nations High Commissioner for refugees field employees. *Journal of Travel Medicine, 8*(3), 117–121.

Raphael, B. (1986). *When Disaster Strikes.* London: Hutchinson.

Sangster, K. (1996). *The role of aid workers in the refugee camp and refugee mass situation.* Unpublished masters thesis, LaTrobe University, Melbourne, Victoria, Australia.

Schouten, E. J., & Borgdorff, M. W. (1995). Increased mortality among Dutch development workers. *British Medical Journal, 311*(7016), 1343–1344.

Segal, D. R., Furukawa, T. P., & Lindh, J. C. (1990). Light infantry as peacekeepers in the Sinai. *Armed Forces & Society, 16*(3), 385–403.

Segal, D. R., Harris, J. J., Rothberg, J. M., & Marlowe, D. H. (1984). Paratroopers as peacekeepers. *Armed Forces & Society, 10*(4), 487–506.

Shakespeare-Finch, J., Paton, D., & Violanti, J. M. (2003). The family: Resilience resource and resilience needs. In D. Paton, J. M. Violanti, & L. Smith. (Eds.), *Promoting Capabilities to Manage Posttraumatic Stress: Perspectives on Resilience* (pp. 170–185). Springfield, IL: Charles C Thomas.

Sharp, T. W., DeFraites, R. F., Thornton, S. A., Burans, J. P., & Wallace, M. R. (1995). Illness in journalists and relief workers involved in international humanitarian assistance efforts in Somalia, 1992–1993. *Journal of Travel Medicine, 2*(2), 70–76.

Sheik, M., Gutierrez, M. I., Bolton, P., Spiegel, P., Thieren, M., & Burnham, G. (2000). Deaths among humanitarian workers. *British Medical Journal, 321,* 166–168.

Shigemura, J., & Nomura, S. (2002). Mental health issues of peacekeeping workers. *Psychiatry & Clinical Neurosciences, 50*(5), 483–491.

Short, P. (1979). Victims and helpers. In R. L. Heathcote, & B. G. Tong (Eds.), *Natural Hazards in Australia.* Canberra: Australian Academy of Science.

Simmonds, S., Gilbert-Miguet, P., Siem, H., Carballo, M., & Zeric, D. (1998). *Occupational Health of Field Personnel in Complex Emergencies: Report of a Pilot Study.* Geneva: World Health Organization.

Smith, B. (2002). The dangers of aid work. In Y. Danieli (Ed.), *Sharing the Front Line and the Back Hills: Peacekeepers, Humanitarian Aid Workers and the Media in the Midst of Crisis* (pp. 171–176). Amityville, NY: Baywood.

Suter, K. (1995, June). *UN peacekeeping operations – what is going wrong?* Paper presented at Auckland University, New Zealand.

Taylor, A. J. W. (1999). Towards the classification of disasters and victims. *Traumatology, 5*(2). Retrieved September 19, 1999, from http://www.fsu.edu/~trauma/

Taylor, A. J. W. (2001). Conflict over the causations of catastrophe. *Australian Journal of Emergency Management, 16*(3), 15–17.

United Nations. (1995). *Tips for Trainers: Stress Management for United States Peacekeepers.* New York: DPKO/Training Unit, p. 37.

van Oudenhoven, J. P., van der Zee, K. I., & van Kooten, M. (2001). Successful adaptation strategies according to expatriates. *International Journal of Intercultural Relations, 25,* 467–482.

Weerts, J. M. P., White, W., Adler, A. B., Castro, C. A., Algra, G., Bramsen, I., et al. (2002). Studies on military peacekeepers. In Y. Danieli (Ed.), *Sharing the Front Line and the Back Hills: Peacekeepers, Humanitarian Aid Workers and the Media in the Midst of Crisis* (pp. 31–48). Amityville, NY: Baywood.

Young, M. A. (2001). *The Community Crisis Response Team Training Manual* (2nd ed.). Washington, DC: National Organization for Victim Assistance.

Chapter 10

WORKING WITH TRAUMA: THE IMPACT ON THE THERAPIST

JACQUIE BICKNELL

INTRODUCTION

For centuries people have rallied to assist others in need. For some, this has become a profession and a career, be it in psychology, social work, psychiatry, counseling, or other disciplines falling under the umbrella of the helping professions. Until recently, however, little attention has been paid to the impact such work/therapeutic engagement could have on the health care professionals involved.

This chapter reviews work conducted over the past decade regarding the experiences of therapists working with clients affected by trauma experiences. The term "therapist" is used to describe health care professionals who regularly engage clients in therapeutic counseling sessions (e.g., psychologists, psychiatrists, social workers, and counselors). This chapter aims to (1) describe positive and negative transformations in therapists in the trauma field, (2) identify risk factors for therapists working in the trauma field, and (3) explore the notion of resilience and growth associated with working in the trauma field.

THERAPIST TRANSFORMATION IN THE TRAUMATOLOGY FIELD

During the past decade traumatology research has increasingly investigated the impact on therapists working with their trauma-affected client base. Research in the late 1980s and early 1990s gained its impetus from anecdotal and supervisory reports of therapists experiencing trauma-based symptoms similar to those experienced and reported by their client base. Since then, trauma therapists, their supervisors, and organizations alike have come to recognize, acknowledge, and/or experience the effects of secondary trauma.

Pioneering work on the negative transformations experienced by therapists was conducted by Herman (1992), Figley (1995), and Pearlman and associates (McCann & Pearlman, 1990; Pearlman & Mac Ian, 1995; Pearlman & Saakvitne, 1995a, 1995b), who write on compassion fatigue (CF) and vicarious trauma (VT), respectively. Another prominent worker in this field is Stamm (1995, 2002) who codeveloped the Compassion Satisfaction Fatigue Practitioner Self-Test (CSF) with Figley (1995). Their work provided the foundation for investigating and managing changes associated with trauma work (Vicary, Searle, & Andrews, 2000).

So far, the research on the negative transformation that occurs for individuals exposed to trauma has been replicated for therapists who engage trauma clients. There also exists a growing literature regarding individuals who experience positive transformations posttrauma. As yet, however, there is no corresponding research on whether a parallel exists for therapists exposed to secondary or vicarious trauma.

Negative Transformations Associated with Trauma Work

The theory of CF presents the impact of trauma therapy as paralleling posttraumatic stress disorder (PTSD). Hence, CF is described as symptomatology of (1) intrusions (e.g., flashbacks, recollections, dreams), (2) avoidance (e.g., avoiding thoughts/feeling, avoiding activities, detachment from others, diminished affect), and (3) hyperarousal (e.g., difficulty staying/falling asleep, hypervigilance, and irritability). The theory of VT, on the other hand, views the negative transformations experienced by trauma therapists as occurring across time and across helping relationships. VT focuses on the disruptions to therapists' (1) frame of reference, (2) capacity to tolerate affect, (3) central needs and beliefs about themselves and others, (4) ego resources, and (5) sensory memory system.

Because of the absence of specialized measures, earlier quantitative research into the phenomenon of secondary trauma drew on instruments typically used with trauma survivor populations designed to measure PTSD, distress levels, and psychopathology (e.g., the Impact of Events Scale [IES], Symptoms Checklist-90 [SCL-90], General Health Questionnaire [GHQ]). More recent research has used specifically designed measures such as the CSF (Stamm & Figley, 1996) and the TSI Belief Scale (Trauma Stress Institute, 1994), a measure of disturbed beliefs considered indicative of secondary trauma (Betts Adams, Matto, & Harrington, 2001; Brady, Guy, Poelstra, & Brokaw, 1999; Pearlman & Mac Ian, 1995; Schauben & Frazier, 1995; van Minnen & Keijsers, 2000). Consistently, studies that have combined quantitative and qualitative investigations of secondary trauma have found greatest support for the phenomenon in the qualitative component of their research. More recent studies, such as Betts Adams et al. (2001), Brady et al. (1999), van Minnen and Keijsers (2000), however, have found differing support for the concept of secondary trauma.

A study by van Minnen and Keijsers (2000), which is the only research so far to compare trauma therapists and nontrauma therapists, found qualitative support for the concept of secondary trauma. In their study, trauma therapists more regularly reported changes of cognition due to trauma work than did their nontrauma colleagues. Quantitatively, however, no significant differences were found between the two therapist groups (trauma n = 20, nontrauma n = 19) as measured by the TSI, SCL-90 and the World Assumptions Scale (WAS) (Janoff-Bulman, 1989).

Although research has identified that secondary trauma may occur once therapists are exposed to trauma work, it is also apparent that not all therapists report trauma work as having a negative impact. This fact prompts the questions: "What can we learn from therapists who appear to engage trauma clients with no or minimal negative effects from their exposure to trauma work?" and "What might be learned from therapists who appear to grow or thrive from their involvement with trauma work?"

Positive Transformations Associated with Trauma Work

Concurrent with the interest in secondary trauma, a paradigm shift has been occurring within psychology and related disciplines. Essentially, there is a call for the focus to swing from deficit-based models, which focus on the pathology presented by individuals, to one where the unexpected success, growth, resilience, and thriving of individuals in the face of adversity are examined. Ickovics and Park (1998) define thriving as "the effective mobilisation of individual and social resources in response to risk or threat, leading to positive mental or physical outcomes and/or positive social outcomes," and further, they argue that "thriving represents something more than a return to equilibrium (i.e., homeostasis) following a challenge" (p. 237). Tedeschi, Park and Calhoun (1998) propose that posttraumatic growth (PTG) explains the process involved as individuals triumph over adversity and consequently grow. They note that PTG manifests in one or more of three key areas: (1) perceptions of self, (2) interpersonal relationships, and (3) philosophy of life.

Similarly, the impetus in the coping literature has swung from a focus on negative affect to one where the role and function of positive affect in stress and well-being is being explored (Folkman & Moskowitz, 2000). Folkman and Moskowitz argue that positive affect can co-occur with distress, that it has an important adaptive function, and that meaning making is significant in promoting and maintaining positive affect during times of distress. The view that positive and negative affects may both coexist and represent a possibly important adaptive function for coping may offer particular insights for the experiences of trauma therapists who endeavor to sustain themselves in work that can both challenge and permanently alter their world. Stamm (2002) queries whether or not a therapist could be at high risk for experiencing CF yet concomitantly be experiencing high compassion satisfaction. Stamm's line of inquiry is consistent with the exploration currently unfolding in the area of coping research that is investigating the significance of positive affect in relation to stress and distress (Folkman & Moskowitz, 2000). As yet, there is no answer to Stamm's query. Early research indicators within the traumatology field, however, suggest that positive affect, satisfaction, or similar concepts may play an important role in therapists' capacity to function effectively when working with trauma clients (Bicknell, 1999; Brady et al., 1999; Steed & Bicknell, 2001; van Minnen & Keijsers, 2000).

RISK FACTORS FOR SECONDARY TRAUMA IN TRAUMA THERAPISTS

Earlier studies focused on exposure and personal trauma history as key predictors of secondary trauma (Pearlman & Mac Ian, 1995; Schauben & Frazier, 1995). Seeking to extend this work and to clarify the relationships between personal and work variables associated with secondary trauma, Betts Adams et al. (2001) found that therapists reporting VT (as measured by the TSI) tend to be younger and have lower annual salaries than therapists with lower TSI scores. Higher scores on the TSI were also associated with more somatic symptoms, a self-perception of less social support, and higher burnout scores. Exposure (number of hours spent with trauma clients and the number of years in trauma work) and personal trauma history were not found to be significant predictors of high TSI scores.

A study by Betts Adams et al. (2001) highlights and represents the complexity of variables that may contribute to secondary trauma and the ambiguity of their causal ordering. Brady et al. (1999) sought clarification of exposure in relation to secondary trauma. Their study of 446 female therapists concluded that (1) current exposure to trauma work, (2) cumulative exposure to trauma work, and (3) intensity of exposure to trauma (i.e., the perceived level of graphic detail disclosed by clients) all contributed significantly to respondents' PTSD-like symptoms (as measured by the IES). Exposure to trauma (current, cumulative, or intensity), however, was not significantly related to therapists' TSI scores. Consequently, Brady et al. (1999) concluded that, while therapists with higher levels of exposure to trauma experience significantly more trauma symptoms themselves, they do not experience significantly more disruption to their cognitive schemas as measured by the TSI. Table 10-1 provides a general framework summarizing the areas theorized as potential risks for therapists (Pearlman & Saakvitne, 1995a, 1995b). It is the interaction between characteristics specific to the therapist and

TABLE 10-1
POTENTIAL RISK FACTORS ASSOCIATED WITH THE DEVELOPMENT OF
SECONDARY TRAUMA IN THERAPISTS

Personal	Professional	Organizational
• Self/personality • Personal history • Current personal circumstances	• Dynamics of the therapeutic process • Level of professional development • Client characteristics • Specific facts of the clients' trauma/abuse/assault	• Organizational contextual factors • Organizational culture • Social/political/cultural issues

his/her situation (professional and organizational issues) that is believed to be significant in the development of secondary trauma for the therapist (Pearlman & Saakvitne, 1995a, 1995b).

Personal Factors (Self/Personality, Personal History, Current Personal Circumstances)

Of the personal factors listed above, personal history appears to be the issue that has received the greatest research attention to date. The discrepant findings, however, highlight the difficulties of concluding that trauma history, per se, is a risk factor for trauma therapists. Several studies (Follette, Polusny, & Milbeck, 1994; Kassam-Adams, 1995; Pearlman & Mac Ian, 1995) have indicated that a childhood history of abuse/trauma is associated with reports of secondary trauma by therapists, whereas others studies (Betts Adams et al., 2001; Brady et al., 1999; Oliveri & Waterman, 1993; Schauben & Frazier, 1995) have not, possibly because of variations in defining what constitutes personal trauma. Studies that have tightened the definition of therapist personal trauma to childhood or adulthood experiences of sexual abuse, rape, a violent crime, or witnessing violence (Betts Adams et al., 2001) and to attempted rape and other childhood or adult sexual harassment (Schauben & Frazier, 1995) have failed to find personal trauma as a predictor of secondary trauma in therapists.

It is possible, therefore, that rather than the personal abuse history per se being the significant factor, whether or not the therapist has addressed this issue may, in fact, be more salient. For example, although not requested in Bicknell's (1999) study, some therapists disclosed and discussed their own experiences of abuse. One therapist disclosed victimization and how that had been managed during trauma work:

> As I had been abused as a child, I sought therapy to help me deal with situations that trigger memories. However, as I had had much therapy before, I've found this rarely impacts on me. I sometimes get "sucked in" by offenders who remind me of my abuser, but I monitor this carefully in supervision. I've found it crucial to be open and honest with my supervisor (Bicknell, 1999, p. 38).

Another therapist wrote of choosing to withdraw from this work for a year and a half because family members had disclosed sexual victimization. Similarly, another therapist chose to seek personal therapy regarding sexual violence she had witnessed during childhood. She indicated that she sought therapy to address issues "mainly around the anger it aroused in me" (Bicknell, 1999, p. 38). Of the therapists who did indicate issues relating to personal experiences of abuse (either as the victim or associated with a significant other), their corresponding risk of CF, as measured using the CSF, was either moderate or less. Hence, it would appear that, although a history of personal trauma may have occurred, therapists are reporting that it rarely effects their adult work as therapists and, on those occasions when it does, they are seeking assistance (i.e., supervision).

Elliot and Guy's (1993) study of 2963 female professionals (340 of whom were mental health professionals) lends support for the view that it is the therapist's resolution of childhood issues, rather than the occurrence thereof, that is important. For example, they found significantly higher incidences of childhood trauma in their sample group of mental health professionals yet higher levels of functioning in adulthood (i.e., less anxiety, depression, dissociation, sleep disturbance, and impairment in their interpersonal relationships) compared with other female professionals. Hence, recording the occurrence of problematic childhood experiences without investigating the therapist's current progress/stage in addressing his/her abuse/trauma could result in the research inconsistencies seen to date and, moreover, suggests caution when concluding that a history of childhood abuse is a significant risk factor for secondary trauma in therapists.

Although current personal circumstances are noted in theories as influential in the development and probable maintenance/exacerbation of secondary trauma (Figley, 1995; Pearlman & Saakvitne, 1995a, 1995b), there is a paucity of research examining the interaction between therapists' current circumstances and secondary trauma. It would be particularly enlightening to examine the interaction and directional nature of the relationship between current circumstances and secondary trauma. I suspect that a bidirectional relationship exists whereby therapists' personal circumstances are both influenced by and influence their experiences of secondary trauma.

Of interest, although empathy is identified as fundamental to the potential development of secondary trauma, neither empathy nor other personal qualities or characteristics of therapists have received much research attention to date. Similarly, the personality factors identified as risk or protective factors for individuals who have experienced trauma are yet to be investigated within therapist populations.

Professional Factors (Dynamics of the Therapeutic Process, Level of Professional Development, Client Characteristics, Specific Facts of Clients' Trauma/Abuse/Assault)

With regard to professional factors, the most attention has been given to the area of professional development that, more often than not, appears to have become entangled with the notion of therapist level of experience or, alternatively, exposure. For example, qualification level is sometimes erroneously equated to more experience in terms of years spent as a therapist. Consistent throughout the literature, however, is recognition of the vulnerability of therapists newest to the field of trauma work, regardless of qualification level or discipline (Betts Adams et al., 2001; Bicknell, 1999; Neuman & Gamble, 1995; Pearlman & Mac Ian 1995; Steed & Bicknell, 2001).

The role and function of supervision (as relevant to professional development) is also theorized as an important mediating factor in the development of secondary trauma, but, as yet, research has not targeted supervision specifically, despite often gathering such information in participant demographics (Neuman & Gamble, 1995; Pearlman & Saakvitne, 1995a, 1995b). The one exception has been van Minnen and Keijsers' (2000) qualitative study comparing trauma and nontrauma therapists. They found that trauma therapists in their sample were less likely than nontrauma therapists to access supervision. Of particular concern was their finding that it was the less experienced trauma therapists who were least likely to receive supervision (i.e., 17 (85%) of a possible 20 therapists did not receive supervision). Comparatively, approximately 35% (i.e., 7/19) of nontrauma therapists did not receive supervision. Reasons cited by trauma therapists for not seeking supervision were represented by one of van Minnen and Keijsers' (2000) sample who stated that "supervision in an official group setting [is] too unsafe an environment in which to talk about personal problems arising from work" (p. 193). Alternatively therapists regarded themselves as having had sufficient experience and therefore no longer requiring supervision or believed that supervision was too time-consuming or expensive. Certainly, notable writers in the field (Figley, 1995; Pearlman & Saakvitne, 1995a, 1995b; Stamm, 1995) highlight the importance of seeking appropriate supervision and not working in isolation when doing trauma work. Again, the quality and expertise of the supervision and therapist amenability to exploring issues associated with secondary trauma may be mediating factors that need to be addressed further.

The very nature of trauma work itself is considered to be a risk factor because it is through this work that therapists are exposed to trauma material. Indeed, the issue of *exposure*, along with the capacity for empathy, is highlighted by both Figley (1995) and Pearlman and associates (McCann & Pearlman, 1990; Pearlman & Mac Ian, 1995; Pearlman & Saakvitne, 1995a, 1995b) as an issue central to their respective theories of CF and VT. Again, however, there is a disparity in the findings relating to the degree of therapist exposure to trauma-associated material. For example, Follette et al. (1994) found that the percentage of caseloads relating to sexual abuse was not significant in predicting secondary trauma, whereas Kassam-Adams (1995), Schauben and Frazier (1995), and Pearlman and Mac Ian (1995) did. As with the issue of "personal abuse history," the concept, and hence the measurement, of exposure may have differed between studies. For example, exposure to trauma-based material could vary according to (1) the amount of time per week spent working with trauma-based material, (2) the overall amount of time exposed to trauma-based material (i.e., how long has the therapist been involved in trauma work), or (3) the perceived intensity or severity of the trauma impact.

In a study of 446 female therapists, Brady et al. (1999) differentiated between subjective distress, particularly posttraumatic stress symptomatology as measured by the IES, and vicarious trauma as measured by the TSI, which is considered to be sensitive to changes in cognitive schemas. While Brady et al. concurred with earlier research that higher exposure corresponded to higher levels of therapist distress, their study also revealed that the more the exposure to trauma material, the higher the therapists' sense of spiritual well-being. Their finding that higher TSI scores were associated with increases in spirituality is interesting because disruption to spirituality, which is considered a key indicator of VT, was conversely considered as a strength and growth area for trauma therapists in the study by Brady et al.

Novice therapists are particularly vulnerable to the effects of secondary trauma. Recommendations are consistently made regarding the importance of educating trauma therapists about the possibility of secondary trauma and normalizing the potential negative impacts of trauma work during supervision with supervisors experienced in trauma work (Betts Adams et al., 2001; Bicknell, 1999; Neuman & Gamble, 1995;

Pearlman & Saakvitne, 1995a, 1995b). It is now well established that, developmentally, therapists are most vulnerable to anxiety in their early years of therapeutic work (Bischoff, Barton, Thober, & Hawley, 2002; Skovholt, 2001), the stage that is typically associated with self-perceptions of therapist competency. It would appear, however, that entry into trauma work may exacerbate competency and identity issues for new therapists and may, in fact, create competency anxiety or an unsettling effect for even seasoned therapists who encounter trauma work (en masse) for the first time in their careers (Bicknell, 1999).

Bischoff's (1997) pilot study of the first three months of therapist-client contact revealed that developing confidence was the primary active developmental process for beginning therapists. He identified that the development of an internal gauge, by which therapists could evaluate their clinical experiences, and the development of boundaries around the self as a helper were the two interrelated processes that supported therapists' development of confidence in the early stages of practice. Subsequently, Bischoff et al. (2002) investigated the external events and experiences influential in the development of clinical self-confidence during graduates' first year of client contact. Their qualitative study, involving 39 graduates from a Marriage and Family Therapy master's degree program (F = 34, M = 5), revealed four themes that affected therapist confidence. Supervision, contact with clients, contact with peers, and personal life stress were considered to be instrumental in the internalization of clinical experiences that leads to the development of a foundation of past clinical experiences with which current clinical experiences can be compared. The first three, supervision, client, and peer contact, could exert either a positive or a negative impact on therapist confidence. Personal life stress, on the other hand, was typically found to affect therapists negatively, essentially distracting them and disrupting the development of clinical experience with which to compare subsequent clinical practice. Considering the above, van Minnen & Keijsers' (2000) finding that it was the least experienced trauma therapists who were choosing not to access supervision is of concern in monitoring the potential for secondary trauma during the early years of trauma work.

Therapist confidence and competence also featured strongly in Bicknell's (1999) qualitative study in which therapists described how entry into trauma work confronted their sense of competency and identity as therapists. New therapists in particular were inclined to keep concerns and vulnerabilities to themselves, fearing others (therapists, supervisors, management) would appraise them as less than capable in their work. The apparent need by therapists early in their trauma work to present themselves as a "got-it-together professionals" was a strong theme in Bicknell's study. That therapists, new therapists in particular, are inclined to withdraw and withhold the impact their work is having on them is concerning and contrary to the implementation of effective measures/strategies to prevent or minimize the potential negative impact of trauma work. Unfortunately, therapist withdrawal or minimal disclosure runs counter to the recommendations for minimizing the possibility of secondary trauma. Essentially, therapist withdrawal provides an opening for the establishment of an unhealthy work dynamic whereby the novice therapist, who is typically eager to do well and be perceived by others, including their supervisors, as competent, is reluctant to discuss the more personal cognitive and affective impact of trauma work. Given the importance of normalizing the impact of the work in order to prevent the onset or development of negative transformations associated with trauma work, such dynamics have the potential to undermine the effective functioning of a trauma workplace and provide a work environment ripe for secondary trauma.

Little appears to have materialized in the research literature regarding factors such as the dynamics of the therapy process or client characteristics. As factors, however, they clearly make intuitive sense in their contribution to secondary trauma and no doubt resonate strongly with trauma therapists and their supervisors alike.

Organizational Factors (Organizational/Contextual Factors, Organizational Culture, Social/Political/Cultural Issues)

As factors contributing to secondary trauma, the organizational factors theorized by Pearlman and Saakvitne (1995a, 1995b) as relevant to the potential development of secondary trauma are yet to receive specific research attention within trauma research. However, drawing from the existing literature, issues of supervision, orientation or integration of new therapists, and what Bicknell (1999) identified as "systems issues" suggest the important role that the organizational setting, culture, and philosophy has on therapists in the trauma field. As already noted, the capacity of an organization to generate a culture that is accepting and normalizing of the potential for negative transformations associated with trauma work is critical for both new and experienced therapists alike. The role of supervision in this regard was discussed above, but other "organizational" issues deserve consideration.

Bicknell (1999) identified "systems issues" as a theme that warranted attention with regard to secondary trauma. Six percent of respondents in her study considered "system issues" to be important in their early stages of trauma work. Representative comments included, "angry at boss, colleague, for lack of empathy for new worker," "trauma, lack of supervision and lack of support," "good supervision got me through."

It would appear that, with time, trauma therapists may experience disillusionment with the system (Bicknell, 1999). For example, one therapist commented,

> I was hoping that there might be space to discuss "parallel process" that occurs in agencies dealing with abuse – that is the abuse dynamics entering the agency, both between staff and between staff and clients. I find this the greatest source of stress and burnout (Bicknell, 1999, p. 45).

Another therapist commented,

> If it was just clients and significant others we were dealing with, the work would be fine. The usual pressures of an insensitive bureaucracy/management, petty professional jealousies, and way over-blown egos contribute far more to the stress levels experienced by workers in this area (Bicknell, 1999, p. 45).

And another described "a sense of frustration as an increasing level of bureaucracy limits effectiveness of treatment programs" (Bicknell, 1999, p. 45). Such comments reflect therapists' growing frustrations and observations of work cultures and dynamics that appear characteristic of trauma work (Herman, 1992; Pearlman & Saakvitne, 1995a, 1995b) and presumably operate to either deplete therapists' reserves and resources and/or serve to distract them from the work they are employed to do.

THERAPIST GROWTH AND RESILIENCE IN TRAUMA WORK

To date research relating to trauma therapists has focused almost exclusively on the negative transformations that may be associated with trauma work, the process by which the transformation may occur, and the factors (personal, professional and organizational) that may be associated with the development of or vulnerability to secondary trauma.

Although evidence of proactive prevention and treatment of secondary trauma exists (Figley, 1995; Pearlman & Saakvitne, 1995a, 1995b; Stamm, 1995), what sustains therapists or contributes to their resilience in trauma work is yet to be established empirically. An area of research that may assist our understanding of potential positive transformations for therapists in trauma work may be drawn from research on resilience, thriving, and posttraumatic growth experienced by individuals who have experienced trauma.

Extending earlier models of resilience, Tedeschi et al. (1998) suggest that posttraumatic growth (PTG) is both an outcome and a process by which the outcome is achieved. Calhoun and Tedeschi (1998) state that, "to account for PTG, it is important to be able to account for how beliefs, goals, identity, and interpersonal behaviour change as the result of stiff challenges to pre-existing patterns in these areas" (p. 222). Calhoun and Tedeschi (1998) indicate that the development of the PTG model was influenced by the literature on (1) the process of change in fundamental beliefs (Janoff-Bulman, 1992), (2) changes in major life goals (McIntosh, 1996; Rothbaum, Weisz & Snyder, 1982; Carver & Scheier, in press, as cited in Tedeschi et al., 1998), (3) identity change (McCann & Pearlman, 1990), and (4) a multitude of works and theories with respect to changes in interpersonal relationships and behavior. Calhoun and Tedeschi (1998) note that fundamental to their model is the understanding that trauma seriously challenges the individual, which results in their reviewing, retaining, expelling, incorporating, and acquiring changes to beliefs, goals, and behaviors. I propose that a process similar to that outlined for PTG may be applicable to therapists exposed to trauma work.

Essentially the PTG model details the growth process experienced by an individual following exposure to a traumatic event. The model proposes that the individuals most likely to move through a growth process have a history of general well-being and exhibit a variety of characteristics that are conducive to growth and development (i.e., a nascent schema encompassing a "complex, active, open and hopeful cognitive style" [Calhoun & Tedeschi, 1998, p. 221]). Exposure to a traumatic event that is of sufficient significance to challenge and alter the individual's world view, fundamental beliefs, values, and so on results in a period of rumination which appears to be more automatic than deliberate in the early stages of change. The focus of this first period of rumination is affect and typically results in emotion-focused coping. The second period of rumination is the reverse whereby rumination appears more deliberate, is primarily cognitive, and correspondingly results in an emphasis on problem-focused coping. Each rumination process reflects the review and relinquishing of long-held beliefs, values, and behaviors that may no longer be applicable, effective, or adaptive.

Hence, in the first instance the individual faces affective challenges, loss, grief, and the task of managing emotional distress. By, and during the second stage of rumination, the emphasis has shifted to a cognitive orientation as individuals disengage from long-held goals, beliefs, and behaviors and begin considering, reviewing, and actioning new ways of coping. Throughout this entire process there is an exchange between the individual and respective support network for support, new ideas, and feedback on changes. The outcome of this process is growth in one or more of the areas indicated. According to Tedeschi et al. (1998), growth is not possible until current coping resources are exhausted, thus allowing new strategies and ways of being to emerge. The growth and wisdom that occurs for some therapists following trauma are eventually achieved when the event and the process have been internalized and incorporated into the individual's life story.

Existing research has shown that trauma therapists can and do change because of their exposure to trauma work. Whether or not therapists experience positive change or growth associated with their exposure to trauma work is yet to be determined. However, within the literature on trauma therapists, factors that are thought to be associated with growth for individuals posttrauma are being identified. For example, earlier research by Schauben and Frazier (1995) indicated that social support (a factor in the PTG model) was important to trauma therapists. The notion of positive spiritual changes also featured in Brady et al.'s (1999) study of trauma therapists. As yet, factors identified in the general population as contributing to Tedeschi et al.'s (1998) concept of a nascent personality (i.e., amenability to change and growth) are yet to be explored in research with trauma therapists.

CONCLUSION

For some therapists, the notion of secondary trauma clearly resonates strongly as a consequence of their transformative experiences. Research has sought to identify predictors of the negative transformations that may be experienced by trauma therapists. Exposure to trauma work and therapist history of personal trauma are the two factors receiving greatest attention to date. More recently, however, research has revealed issues indicative of positive transformations, such as social support and spirituality. Understanding the nature of the relationship between protective factors such as social support and spirituality and trauma therapists' experiences in the trauma field may assist our understanding of how therapists sustain themselves while working in the trauma field.

The latter part of this chapter raised the possibility of therapist resilience or growth associated with trauma work. Although there is still much to be understood regarding the factors contributing to secondary trauma, especially professional and organizational factors, I suggest that research in the area of therapist resilience and potential growth associated with trauma work has much to offer our field. Hopefully research with trauma therapists will soon reflect the research emphasis emerging elsewhere, and we will begin to gain an empirical understanding of what sustains trauma therapists in their workplace.

REFERENCES

Betts Adams, K., Matto, H. C., & Harrington, D. (2001). The Traumatic Stress Institute Belief Scale as a measure of vicarious trauma in a national sample of clinical social workers. *Families in Society: The Journal of Contemporary Human Services, 82*, 363–371.

Bicknell, J. (1999). *Trauma and the therapist: The experience of therapists working with the perpetrators of sexual abuse.* Unpublished honour's dissertation, Curtin University of Technology, Perth, Western Australia, Australia.

Bischoff, R. J. (1997). Themes in therapist development during the first three months of clinical experience. *Contemporary Family Therapy, 19*, 563–580.

Bischoff, R. J., Barton, M., Thober, J., & Hawley, R. (2002). Events and experiences impacting the development of clinical self confidence: A study of the first year of client contract. *Journal of Marital and Family Therapy, 28*(3), 371–382.

Brady, J. L., Guy, J. D., Poelstra, P. L., & Brokaw, B. F. (1999). Vicarious traumatization, spirituality, and the treatment of sexual abuse survivors: A national survey of women psychotherapists. *Professional Psychology: Research and Practice, 30*(4), 386–393.

Calhoun, L. G., & Tedeschi, R. G. (1998). Posttraumatic growth: Future directions. In R. G. Tedeschi, C. L. Park, & L. G. Calhoun (Eds.), *Posttraumatic Growth: Positive Changes in the Aftermath of Crisis* (pp. 215–238). New Jersey: Lawrence Erlbaum.

Elliot, D. M., & Guy, J. D. (1993). Mental health professionals versus non-mental-health professionals: Childhood trauma and adult functioning. *Professional Psychology: Research and Practice, 24*(1), 83–90.

Figley, C. (1995). *Compassion Fatigue. Coping with Secondary Traumatic Stress Disorder in Those Who Treat the Traumatised.* New York: Brunner/Mazel.

Folkman, S., & Moskowitz, J. T. (2000). Positive affect and the other side of coping. *American Psychologist, 55*(6), 647–654.

Follette, V. M., Polusny, M. M., & Milbeck, K. (1994). Mental health and law enforcement professionals: Childhood trauma and adult functioning. *Professional Psychology: Research and Practice, 15* 833–845.

Herman, J. L. (1992). Trauma and Recovery: *The Aftermath of Violence from Domestic Abuse to Political Terror.* New York: Basic Books.

Ickovics, J. R., & Park, C. L. (1998). Paradigm shift: Why a focus on health is important. *Journal of Social Issues, 54*(2), 237–244.

Janoff-Bulman, R. (1989). Assumptive worlds and the stress of traumatic events: Applications of the schema-construct. *Social Cognition, 7,* 113–136.

Janoff-Bulman, R. (1992). *Shattered Assumptions.* New York: The Free Press.

Kassam-Adams, N. (1995). The risks of treating sexual trauma: Stress and secondary trauma among therapists. In B. Stamm (Ed.), *Secondary Traumatic Stress: Self-care Issues for Clinicians, Researchers, and Educators* (pp. 37–50). Maryland: Sidran Press.

McCann, I. L., & Pearlman, L. A. (1990). Vicarious traumatization: A framework for understanding the psychological effects of working with victims. *Journal of Traumatic Stress, 3,* 131–149.

McIntosh, W. D. (1996). When does goal nonattainment lead to negative emotional reaction, and when doesn't it?: The role of linking and rumination. In L. L. Martin & A. Tesser (Eds.), *Striving and Feeling: Interactions among Goals, Affect, and Self-regulation* (pp. 53–77). Mahwah, NJ: Lawrence Erlbaum.

Neumann, D. A., & Gamble, S. J. (1995). Issues in the professional development of psychotherapists: Countertransference and vicarious traumatization in the new trauma therapists. *Psychotherapy, 32,* 341–347.

O'Leary, V. E. (1998). Strength in the face of adversity: Individual and social thriving. *Journal of Social Issues, 54*(2), 425–446.

O'Leary, V. E., & Ickovics, J. R. (1995). Resilience and thriving in response to challenge: An opportunity for a paradigm shift in women's health. *Women's Health: Research on Gender, Behaviour and Policy, 1,* 121–142.

Oliveri, M. K., & Waterman, J. (1993). Impact on therapists. In J. Waterman, R. K. Kelly, M. K. Oliveri, & J. McCord. (Eds.), *Behind the Playground Walls: Sexual Abuse in Preschools* (pp. 190–202). New York: Guilford Press.

Pearlman, L. A., & Mac Ian, P. S. (1995). Vicarious traumatization: An empirical study of the effects of trauma work on trauma therapists. *Professional Psychology: Research and Practice, 26,* 558–565.

Pearlman, L. A., & Saakvitne, K. W. (1995a). *Trauma and the Therapists: Countertransference and Vicarious Traumatization in Psychotherapy with Incest Survivors.* New York: Norton.

Pearlman, L. A., & Saakvitne, K. W. (1995b). Treating therapists with vicarious traumatization and Secondary Traumatic Stress Disorder. In C. R. Figley (Ed.), *Compassion Fatigue: Coping with Secondary Traumatic Stress Disorder in Those Who Treat the Traumatised* (pp. 150–177). New York: Brunner/Mazel.

Rothbaum, F., Weisz, J. R., & Snyder, S. S. (1982). Changing the world and changing the self: A two-process model of perceived control. *Journal of Personality and Social Psychology, 42*, 5–37.

Schauben, L. J., & Frazier, P. A. (1995). Vicarious trauma: The effects on female counselors of working with sexual violence survivors. *Psychology of Women Quarterly, 19*, 49–64.

Skovholt, T. M. (2001). *The Resilient Practitioner: Burnout Prevention and Self-care Strategies for Counselors, Therapists and Health Professionals.* Sydney: Allyn and Bacon.

Stamm, B. H. (Ed.). (1995). *Secondary Traumatic Stress: Self-care Issues for Clinicians, Researchers, and Educators.* Lutherille, MD: Siridan Press.

Stamm, B. H. (2002). Measuring compassion satisfaction as well as fatigue: Developmental history of the Compassion Satisfaction and Fatigue Test. In C. R. Figley (Ed.), *Treating Compassion Fatigue* (pp. 107–119). New York: Taylor & Francis.

Stamm, B. H., & Figley, C. R. (1996). *Compassion Satisfaction and Fatigue Test.* Retrieved May 17, 2002, from http://www.isu.edu/~bhstamm/tests.html

Steed, L., & Bicknell, J. (2001). Trauma and the therapist: The experience of therapists working with the perpetrators of sexual abuse. *The Australasian Journal of Disaster and Trauma Studies-E, 2.* Retrieved May 24, 2002, from http://www.massey.ac.nz/%7Etrauma/issues/2001-1

Tedeschi, R. G., & Calhoun, L. G. (1996). The Posttraumatic Growth Inventory: Measuring the positive legacy of trauma. *Journal of Traumatic Stress, 9*, 455–471.

Tedeschi, R. G., Park. C. L., & Calhoun, L. G. (1998). *Posttraumatic Growth: Positive Changes in the Aftermath of Crisis.* New Jersey: Lawrence Erlbaum.

Traumatic Stress Institute. (1994). *The TSI Belief Scale.* South Windsor, CT: TSI.

van Minnen, A., & Keijsers, G. P. J. (2000). A controlled study into the (cognitive) effects of exposure treatment on trauma therapists. *Journal of Behaviour Therapy and Experimental Psychiatry, 31*, 189–200.

Vicary, D., Searle, G., & Andrews, H. (2000). Assessment and intervention with Kosovar refugees: Design and management of a therapeutic team. *The Australasian Journal of Disaster and Trauma Studies-E, 2.* Retrieved June 27, 2001, from http://www.massey.ac.nz/%7Etrauma/issues/2000-2

Chapter 11

THE PSYCHOLOGICAL IMPACT
OF WORK ORGANIZATION

PETER SEVASTOS

INTRODUCTION

The workplace at the beginning of the 21st century finds itself with challenges unequaled in the history of the organization of work. The globalization of markets, changes in the political and legal and industrial relations systems, privatization, demographic changes, technological advances, and a shift in emphasis away from manufacturing industries toward the delivery of services (Borland, Gregory, & Sheehan, 2001), have all contributed to an increasingly uncertain work environment.

To meet the demands of this new order, organizations have had to find new ways to manage their workforce through organizational restructuring such as downsizing, the creation of leaner and flatter structures, the introduction of new forms of work redesigns, and the intensification of work by the adoption of flexible employment practices. Pressures for flexibility are not only in response to competition due to market forces but also from customers and shareholders. Inevitably, these measures have increased the demands of work, inequality in income distribution, and the physical and psychological health risks associated with them. Consequently, organizations must attend not only to the prevention of physical hazards in the workplace but also to the identification and control of organizational factors that contribute to poor mental health.

THE NEW WORKPLACE

After more than a decade of organizational restructuring, downsizing, and outsourcing of key organizational functions, there is a genuine concern among workers that their jobs, wages, and working conditions are slowly being eroded (Borland, Gregory, & Sheehan, 2001). The phenomenon of downsizing is pervasive in all Western economies (Dawkins, Littler, Venezuela, & Jensen, 1999). Job classifications affected by these changes were predominantly managers and similar executives. Those who survived the change registered lower levels of commitment, morale, motivation, and higher levels of perceived insecurity.

Organizational restructuring usually follows downsizing. The three-tiered organization – made up of a core of full-time, highly skilled managers and knowledge workers, a layer of permanent part-time, and temporary or casual employees, supplemented by external consultants – is a response to a leaner workforce (Atkinson, 1985). This strategic approach to staffing is aimed at achieving maximum flexibility as a way of controlling labor costs by delivering just-in-time staffing arrangements. It is a growing trend (Dunlop, 2001). The inevitable consequence of the new type of organization is a dramatic reduction of the workforce referred to euphemistically by some commentators as "rightsizing" (Hitt, Keats, Harback, & Nixon, 1994).

A strong association between downsizing and deskilling has been found, supporting the view that valuable skills and knowledge are lost to organizations when they downsize (Dawkins & Littler, 2001). Clay (1998) reports a study by Cascio who, with his colleagues, examined the Standard & Poor 500's performance over a period of 15 years. They discovered that organizations which downsized without introducing other changes never outperformed other companies. Inevitably, downsizing an organization imposes greater demands on the remaining core staff who, in addition to handling the increased workload stemming from the reduction in the number of people employed, have to deal with the supervision of temporary or casual personnel who may lack the necessary skills and knowledge to performs the required tasks.

All of these changes have added to the unpredictability and complexity of working conditions and have contributed to a psychological environment that is increasingly hostile. But how can organizations redress this setback that has been steadily growing over the last few decades and create favorable conditions for the emergence of a better and more fulfilling working life?

As a first step, organizations will need to undertake a thorough evaluation of their work practices and identify the risk factors that effect workers' mental health. The employing organization has a "duty of care" towards its employees "so far as is practicable"; that is, if it is capable of being done, the organization is required to implement policies that will protect workers from hazards and maintain a safe and healthy workplace (WorkSafe, 1999). The word "healthy" could be used in its broader sense and may include not only prevention of physical injuries, but also ailments due to stress if it is shown that the working environment had contributed to them. However, in Australia, the Occupational Health and Safety (OHS) legislation does not mention explicitly psychological hazards in the workplace. A more enlightened approach towards a "healthy" working environment, for example, has been adopted by the Swedish Work Environment Authority (n.d.) through its legislative powers and takes into consideration the mental and social conditions of work:

> Monotony, stress and isolation at work are to be avoided by adapting working conditions to human aptitudes. This again applies to such questions as well-being and satisfaction at work. The aim is for work to be found a meaningful, rewarding aspect of life (Chap. 2).

The discussion that follows identifies the most prevalent risk factors that exist in the new workplace, so that organizational practices and policies may be implemented aimed at protecting the safety and health of workers.

JOB CHARACTERISTICS

Voluminous research supports the hypothesis that job features, such as job demands and the opportunity to exercise decision latitude or control, are closely associated with mental strain (Sauter & Hurrell, 1999). One influential model that received much empirical scrutiny over the last two decades is Karasek's (1979) demand-control model of organizational strain. This model has been instrumental in demonstrating the extent to which certain job characteristics effect the experience of work, and a worker's subsequent well-being, psychological strain, and mental health (Carayon, 1993). Research on blue collar employees (Karasek,

1979), white collar employees (Bourbonnais, Brisson, Moisan, & Vezina, 1996), and European and North American populations (Karasek, 1979) has identified, in addition to various physical health outcomes such as cardiovascular disease (CHD) (Siegrist & Klein, 1990) and myocardial infarction risk (Karasek & Theorell, 1990), psychological outcomes such as depression (Carayon, 1993; Landsbergis, 1988) and other related psychiatric illnesses (Bourbonnais et al., 1996).

The model proposes that jobs vary to the degree that they possess job features that are considered psychologically demanding by workers (e.g., workload, time pressures) and the degree to which the job affords one the opportunity to exercise decision latitude or control over work processes (e.g., participation in decision making). The model further asserts that the extent to which demands exceed control will determine strain, and that this relationship is not only additive, but also interactive in nature; that is, strain is likely to be affected disproportionately when demands exceed opportunities for control. It should be borne in mind, however, that if demands are balanced with opportunities for control, the results are not only positive for the individual in terms of strain outcomes, but they offer, in addition, opportunities for skill utilization and learning. Karasek (1979) labeled the jobs "active."

Subsequently, Karasek, and Theorell (1990) modified the model to include one other work environment characteristic thought to moderate the worker's experience of strain: social support. Indeed, social support, especially from a worker's direct supervisor, has been found to add to the predictive power in explaining health outcomes (Carayon, Yang, & Lee, 1995; Parker & Kulik, 1995; Terry, Nielsen, & Perchard, 1993; Yang & Carayon, 1995).

The demand-control model has been subjected to intense scrutiny, and several criticisms of the model have been presented in the literature, based primarily on measurement and methodological issues (Ganster, 1989; Hurrell & McLaney, 1989; Lubinski & Humphreys, 1990; Spector, 1987). Others (Fletcher & Jones, 1993) also have suggested the incorporation of a wider range of variables that potentially would account for additional variance in the strain outcomes. Warr (1987), for example, proposed a Vitamin Model of psychological health by making job features analogous to vitamins, where the consumption of more is not necessarily better.

The Vitamin Model identifies the following ten environmental features (Warr, 1999): opportunity for personal control (i.e., autonomy), opportunity for skill use (i.e., utilization of valued skills), externally generated goals (i.e., quantitative and qualitative workload), variety (i.e., task variety), environmental clarity (i.e., feedback from the job), availability of money (i.e., income level), physical security (i.e., health and safety), supportive supervision (i.e., supervisory support), opportunity for interpersonal contact (i.e., social interaction), and valued social position (i.e., significance of work). Similar to some vitamins that can have either a beneficial effect (if taken in moderation) or a detrimental effect (if taken in large doses), these environmental features can either promote or decrease psychological health.

Aspects of the environment that have the potential to impair psychological health if they are present beyond a required level are opportunities for personal control, opportunities for skill use, supportive supervision, opportunities for interpersonal contact, variety, environmental clarity, and externally generated goals. Other features, like certain vitamins if taken in large doses, do not appear to have any ill effects. These environmental features include availability of money, physical security, and valued social position. These features increase psychological health up to a point and then level off, maintaining what Warr (1994) terms a "constant effect." Consistent with this model Warr argues that his Vitamin Model of well-being would predict that opportunities for control and skill use (or job decision latitude) would have a curvilinear relationship with well-being. Limited support for Warr's model, based on cross-sectional data sets, has been reported in the literature (Warr, 1990; De Jonge & Schaufeli, 1998).

Warr (1990), rather than predicting additive and interactive relationships between demand, control, and indices of well-being, assumes that a quadratic or curvilinear function would more adequately explain the relationship. Under Warr's Vitamin Model it is assumed that up until a certain level, certain job characteristics, including demands and control, are considered healthy and contribute to the avoidance of job strain. However, when levels of these characteristics, such as demands and support, increase beyond an optimum level for the individual, strain is likely to result simply through overload.

WORK ROLES

Another source of psychological strain is associated with the expectations attached to particular role sets. Given that each organizational role comprises several activities, and that several roles within a role set may be part of a single office, it is not uncommon to find that these organizational roles may be in disagreement with one another. In addition, if these roles are not stated explicitly, as is the case with many managerial and executive jobs, there is great ambiguity as to what is expected from the role.

Role conflict has been defined as "the simultaneous occurrence of two or more role expectations such that compliance with one would make compliance with the other more difficult" (Katz & Kahn, 1978, p. 204). Role ambiguity is "uncertainty about what the occupant of a particular office is supposed to do" (Katz & Kahn, 1978, p. 206). If role conflict, role ambiguity, or both are present within a job at high levels, the individual is likely to suffer from psychological strain (Jackson & Schuler, 1985; Katz & Kahn, 1978; O'Driscoll & Beehr, 2000).

Over recent years, role overload or "the perception that one is being asked to do more than time permits, although the required activities themselves are neither intrinsically incompatible or beyond one's abilities" (Katz, & Kahn, 1978, p. 598) has received more attention due to organizational restructuring and downsizing that resulted in the intensification of work. Quantitative (too much work to complete) rather than qualitative (work that is too complex to do) overload is mainly the experience of those whose organizations have been downsized, resulting in under-utilization of skills and loss of control, especially in white collar jobs (Dawkins & Littler, 2001; Worrall & Cooper, 1998).

In the UK, the USA, and Australia these changes had detrimental consequences for families and communities, not only for those who were displaced, but also for those who survived downsizing (Grunberg, Moore, & Greenberg, 2001; Pocock, 2002). Protective service organizations are not immune to such changes. There seems to be an expectation from management that, even with fewer employees, more work than previously was expected can be accomplished. Downsizing the organization without alleviating the workload and time pressures can manifest itself various dysfunctional consequences for the individual and organization alike (Narayanan, Menon, & Spector, 1999). The negative impact of downsizing may be neutralized, however, if the organization adopts a strategic approach to change by introducing measures that mitigate the effects of increased work demands (Parker, Chmiel, & Wall, 1997). Excessive work demands, often reported through the media, are found predominantly in the services sector including public health, the police, and education (Gillespie, Walsh, Winefield, Dua, & Stough, 2001).

Workload, in particular, has increased among full-time employees in the managerial, professional, and para-professional classifications (Buchanan & van Wanrooy, 2002). These increases in working time have serious implications for the general well-being of employees (Rosa, 1995). In a meta-analytic study, based on quantitative and qualitative reviews of the literature, a clear association was found between hours of work and ill health (Sparks, Cooper, Fried, & Shirom, 1997).

EMOTIONAL LABOR

The service sector of the economy has been growing steadily worldwide over the last few decades, and new interpersonal role requirements are required for service providers. For the period between 1991 and 2001, the global economic activity registered an 18-percent increase in the service sector; during the same period there was a decrease in the agriculture and industry sectors (World Data, 1991, 2001). The technology of service organizations is characterized by the following (Daft, 2001, p. 210):
- Intangible outputs based on knowledge and ideas
- Simultaneous production and consumption (i.e., the product does not exist until it is requested by a client)
- Labor and knowledge intensive
- High interaction with clients, emphasizing the importance of employees in the delivery of service
- Subjective measurement of quality of output
- Rapid response time
- Location of site for the delivery of service dispersed to meet the demands of clients

The technological characteristics associated with the service sector require knowledge and skills very dissimilar to those of manufacturing organizations that are capital intensive, deal with tangible products that can be inventoried, and have little direct contact with the client (Daft, 2001). The demands made on service providers are also much different because of the emphasis on interpersonal requirements for the delivery of these services. Given the importance of interpersonal skills in service organizations, recent research has sought to identify their predictors.

Emotional intelligence (EI) is one such candidate and has been defined as "the ability to monitor one's own and others' emotions, to discriminate among them, and to use the information to guide one's thinking and action" (Salovey & Mayer, 1990, p. 189). The components of emotional intelligence are self-awareness, self-regulation, motivation, empathy, and social skill (Goleman, 1995). They have performance implications for service providers. For example, self-regulation (i.e., the ability to control one's moods or emotions) is an important dimension in professions that require face-to-face interaction for the effective performance of work (e.g., nurses, police officers, and psychologists). However, such self-regulation, as for example, when the individual is required by the work role to hide negative emotions by faking, may act as a stressor on the individual and lead to undesirable effects because of excessive emotional labor (Brotheridge & Grandey, 2002; Schaubroeck & Jones, 2000).

Emotional labor has been defined as "the effort, planning, and control needed to express organizationally desired emotion during interpersonal transactions" (Morris & Feldman, 1996, p. 987), and it is becoming an increasingly more important contextual job element in the new workplace. However, this job requirement may have undesirable psychological consequences for the service provider (Ahsford & Humphreys, 1993; Wharton & Erickson, 1993). Morris and Feldman (1996) proposed that the greater the requirement to interact face-to-face with a client, the greater the emotional dissonance experienced by the service provider, and that the frequency and variety of emotional display, and the attentiveness to display the rules required, will be positively associated with emotional exhaustion. A recent study involving 1,241 participants found that work requiring emotional labor predicted burnout. For service professionals, the interaction of emotional dissonance with other organizational stressors predicted elevated levels of emotional exhaustion and depersonalization (Zapf, Seifert, Schmutte, Mertini, & Holz, 2001). However, Schaubroeck and Jones (2000) found that only emotional labor that was perceived as inauthentic by the service provider was associated with psychological distress – not the emotional labor itself.

Organizational roles may not simply be the fulfillment of emotional and behavioral expectations vis-à-vis a client or other organizational members. More broadly, it may incorporate a value system of professional conduct that is often at odds with the management of the employing organization. Nearly half a century ago, Gouldner (1957) made the distinction between cosmopolitans and locals to differentiate those organizational members who identify with the values of their profession, as opposed to those whose loyalties lie with the management of the employing organization. Such clashes of values are often reported in the media, e.g., when a hospital medical practitioner opposes the early discharge of patients from hospital imposed by administration due to economic rather than medical considerations. Cost-cutting practices aimed at maximizing efficiencies or questionable ethical standards in the delivery of services (e.g., the accounting firm Arthur Andersen) have the potential to create tension within the individual that leads to psychological distress. In addition, if an employee refuses to perform practices that are incompatible with his or her professional and ethical standards, resists openly, or expresses "civic courage" by becoming a whistle-blower, the consequences are severe. In such situations one could expect retaliation from management, especially if the reported misconduct was systematic or the flawed practices were part of the regular money-making activities of the organization (Rothschild & Miethe, 1999).

JOB INSECURITY

An inevitable consequence of organizational change based on restructuring and downsizing is that surviving employees, especially white-collar and professional employees, experience high levels of job insecurity (Worrall & Cooper, 1998). The concept of a "job for life" is now an anachronism, and the unstated "reciprocal exchange agreement" (Robinson & Rousseau, 1994, p. 246) in the form of a "psychological contract" between the worker and the employing organization has been irrevocably broken.

Job insecurity has been defined as an "overall concern about the future existence of the job" (Rosenblatt & Ruvio, 1996, p. 587) and is experienced by the individual as a stressor (Sverke & Hellgren, 2002). However, job insecurity may also be affected by a change in job content or work environment (Borland, 2001) or even conditions under which the job is carried out (O'Neill, 2002). Using the argument that job insecurity is the price we pay to remain competitive in a global economy, many organizations, in their drive to reduce costs and increase profits, downsized their organizations, creating conditions that are affecting the psychological health of their employees and their families in the process (Burchell et al., 1999).

Several studies have reported the adverse effects of job insecurity. An exploration of the impact of organizational change on the job security of employees following a merger was assessed longitudinally (Probst, 2002). Six months after the merger, study results confirmed that organizational change affected perceptions of job security, and that these changes in perception were related to other organizational variables (e.g., absenteeism). A North American study (Reynolds, 2001) using ordered probit analysis (N = 2,798) confirmed that the traditional sources of insecurity, such as layoffs and seasonal work, are common among the unskilled, those engaged in sales, service, and blue collar occupations, whereas exposure to downsizing is common among white-collar employees. Furthermore, when witnessing organizational downsizing, white-collar employees hold perceptions of the probability of job loss that are higher than those of other workers.

In a study of 336 Belgian metal industry workers, perceptions of job insecurity were associated with lower levels of well-being, after controlling for the effects of gender and age. For those who felt insecure, scores on the General Health Questionnaire-2 (GHQ-2) were no different than scores from a representative sample of short-term unemployed (De-Witte, 1999).

Job insecurity was also investigated in an Australian public transport organization in a comparison of 32 employees in a redundant group with 63 employees in a control group. A marked deterioration in psychological health was detected. Neither support from peers, management, nor unions appeared to protect those experiencing job insecurity, a result consistent with the conclusions of Burchell et al. (1999). Sources of potential support did not have any buffering effect, leading the researchers to conclude that perceptions of job insecurity had to be dealt with directly, rather than relying on the moderating influence of social support to render it less harmful (Dekker & Schaufeli, 1995).

WORKPLACE HARASSMENT AND VIOLENCE

We live in a violent society – a trend evidenced by all industrialized countries. Social deviance in the Australian community increased dramatically during the decade 1989–1999. Reported assaults per 100,000 of the population, for example, increased by 302.6, while burglaries and break-ins increased by 222.2 for the same period (World Data, 1989, 1999). Organizations have not been immune from this trend. Recently, reports of insider trading and the highly publicized corporate failures in Australia of Ansett and HIH insurance resulted in thousands of employees not only losing their jobs but also their financial entitlements. In the USA the collapse of Enron, and the involvement of the accounting firm Arthur Andersen in the cover-up of Enron's true financial position, raised questions of ethical conduct, and, inevitably, an examination of the value system of modern organizations. Within a culture that tolerates social deviance, the individual is often at the mercy of those in power, while a breakdown of community spirit within the organization due to job insecurity and an emphasis on profits rather than people often leads to a clash of values, conflict, and the fragmentation of team work (Maslach & Leiter, 1997). The individual worker is vulnerable to antisocial behaviors not only from managers and fellow-workers in the form of bullying and physical assault, such as sexual harassment, but, increasingly, from the general public. Physical violence by the public toward an employee is frequent in such occupations as nursing and law enforcement.

Workplace violence has been defined by the National Institute for Occupational Safety and Health (NIOSH) (2002a) as "violent acts (including assaults, and threats of assaults) directed towards persons at work or on duty" (p. 5), and it also is expressed in terms of threats (including verbal, written, or symbolic threats to cause harm), physical assaults (ranging from physical contact with or without a weapon), and muggings (aggravated assaults with the intent to rob). Even when an employee is not directly involved in the act of violence, he or she may be psychologically affected by the incident. Workers vulnerable to physical attacks usually work alone or in small groups (e.g., police officers on patrol) and in isolated locations. Workers on duty beyond the normal working day (i.e., beyond 6:00 pm), in particular, are especially vulnerable.

A serious social-relational aspect of work that acts as an organizational stressor is bullying, and it is present when the victim perceives that he or she is "at the receiving end of some form of persistent, harassing hehaviour" (Hoel, Rayner, & Cooper, 1999, p. 218). The type of bullying may vary according to organizational status. In a large UK study (N = 5,288), the results showed that whereas the prevalence of bullying, its duration, and status of the perpetrator were common across all occupational categories, workers and supervisors were more frequently subjected to negative acts directed towards the self (i.e., derogatory or exclusionary behaviors); managers were more frequently exposed to work-related acts such as extreme work pressure (Hoel, Cooper, & Faragher, 2001). That high-status employees are exposed more frequently to negative work-related acts is supported by a study of business professionals whose views about work-related matters were ignored, and who experienced the imposition of unreasonable deadlines and the withholding of information necessary to complete their work (Salin, 2001). The experience of being bullied may lead to psychological trauma. Mikkelsen and Einarsen (2002) examined the prevalence of posttraumatic stress disorder (PTSD) among a group of 118 victims of bullying. They found that 76% of the victims exhibited symptoms of PTSD and suggested that bullying at work may also increase negative views about self, others, and the world in general.

Harassment and any other form of deviant behavior can be controlled by the organization if there is a climate of management intolerance toward such acts. In a recent study that investigated sexual harassment at work, results showed that when organizational leaders were supportive of policies aimed at counteracting these acts, women were significantly freer to report incidents of harassment than when leaders were perceived as being less supportive of these policies (Offermann & Malamut, 2002).

SURVEILLANCE

The prevention and control of hazards at work, both physical and psychological, require a surveillance mechanism, not only at the organizational level, but also at the local government and federal levels. A report produced by the Department of Health and Human Services of the Centers for Disease Control and Prevention (National Institute for Occupational Safety and Health, 2002b) laments the fact that the "capacity to track and describe changing patterns of work is very limited" (p. 5) following the demise in 1977 of the Quality of Employment Survey (QES) that collected systematic data on working conditions. Presently, in the USA, this type of information is obtained through various sources, e.g., the Bureau of Labor Statistics. By contrast, the European Union carries out cross-national surveys on working conditions and the organization of work every five years (National Institute for Occupational Safety and Health, 2002b, p. 5). In Australia information on working conditions is collected by the Australian Bureau of Statistics (ABS) and through research carried out by the Australian Council for Trade Unions (ACTU) at the national level. However, these efforts by the ACTU, even though laudable, are fragmented and lack the systematic approach taken by the European Union. What is required in Australia is a federal initiative to collect survey data on the working environment periodically so that individual organizations can use the results for benchmarking. At present, however, attempts at benchmarking are carried out by individual organizations with the help of external consultancies that use a variety of measures, often psychometrically inadequate, to benchmark their human resources policies.

The position taken in this chapter is that efforts should be directed toward the identification and prevention of psychological hazards in the workplace. It, therefore, concentrates on interventions at the primary level rather than the secondary or tertiary level (Kompier, 1996). Kompier suggests that prevention requires steps to be taken to intervene at the source of the problem (primary level) by modifying the working environment, for example, through the redesign of jobs or through selection procedures aimed at achieving high levels of job-person fit (Edwards & Cooper, 1990; Bretz & Judge, 1994), as opposed to companies' reacting after the event when employees show early signs of psychological distress (secondary level) or when they require rehabilitation through employee assistance programs (EAPs) after sick leave (tertiary level).

Effective preventative measures to identify and control psychological hazards in the workplace presuppose strong commitment from management. However, this commitment can only come about if links can be established between good practices conducive to the physical and mental health of workers and organizational effectiveness. In this regard, organizational psychologists and human resources professionals can assist not only by disseminating research findings on these issues but also by conducting research that uses robust quasi-experimental designs to answer questions of effectiveness (i.e., reduced levels of sick leave and absenteeism, improved quality performance, etc.) stemming from worker health-sensitive policies. To drive such an agenda, Karasek (2001) envisions professionals who combine humane well-being goals from a public health perspective and psychological and sociological wisdom with knowledge of the world of work and its effects on people.

A proactive approach to the management of psychological well-being in the workplace starts with an assessment of health risks. This assessment requires the involvement of occupational health and safety professionals, organizational psychologists, human resources practitioners, and employee representatives from all organizational levels. A participative approach facilitates the formulation of human resources policies, guidelines, and reporting mechanisms. Their implementation requires the careful dissemination of information through training and educational effort.

Identification and assessment of risk require the use of different methodologies for the collection of data, e.g., observational methods, focus groups, interviews, and survey research. Data on job features and indicators of well-being should be collected periodically, preferably biannually. Ideally, individual cases should be matched over time to detect any changes in attitudes and practices, but only if appropriate steps and procedures have been taken to secure confidentiality of respondents. Results of comparisons over time should be widely reported, and they ought to form part of an organization's annual report as an index of performance.

REFERENCES

Ahsford, B. E., & Humphreys, R. H. (1993). Emotional labor in service roles: The influence of identity. *Academy of Management Review, 18,* 88–115.

Atkinson, J. (1985). Flexibility: Planning for an uncertain future. *Manpower Policy and Practice, 1,* 26–29.

Australian Bureau of Statistics. (1999). Year book Australia. *Special article – Casual employment* (ABS catalogue number 6203.0). Canberra: Australian Bureau of Statistics.

Australian Council for Trade Unions. (2002a). *Fifty families. What unreasonable hours are doing to Australians, their families and their communities.* Retrieved from http://actu.labor.net.au/papers/

Australian Council for Trade Unions. (2002b). *ACTU reasonable hours test case affiliates information kit.* Retrieved from http://actu.labor.net.au/papers/

Borland, J. (2001). Job stability and job security. In J. Borland, B. Gregory, & P. Sheehan (Eds.), *Work Rich, Work Poor* (pp. 142–159). Melbourne: Victoria University, Centre for Strategic Economic Studies.

Borland, J., Gregory, B., & Sheehan, P. (Eds.). (2001). *Work Rich, Work Poor.* Melbourne: Victoria University, Centre for Strategic Economic Studies.

Borland, J., Gregory, B., & Sheehan, P. (2001). Inequality and economic change. In J. Borland, B. Gregory, & P. Sheehan (Eds.), *Work Rich, Work Poor* (pp. 1–20). Melbourne: Victoria University, Centre for Strategic Economic Studies.

Bourbonnais, R., Brisson, C., Moisan, J., & Vezina, M. (1996). Job strain and psychological distress in white collar workers. *Scandinavian Journal of Work, Environment, & Health, 22*, 139–145.

Bretz, R. D., & Judge, T. A. (1994). Person-organization fit and the theory of work adjustment: Implications for satisfaction, tenure, and career success. *Journal of Vocational Behavior, 44*, 32–54.

Brotheridge, C. M., & Grandey, A. A. (2002). Emotional labor and burnout: Comparing two perspectives of "people work." *Journal of Vocational Behavior, 60*, 17–39.

Buchanan, J., & van Wanrooy, B. (2002). *What about the Bosses? Employees and Extended Hours of Work.* Melbourne: Australian Council of Trade Unions.

Burchell, B. J., Day, D., Hudson, M., Lapido, D., Mankelow, R., Nolan, J. P., et al. (1999). *Job Insecurity and Work Intensification. Flexibility and the Changing Boundaries of Work.* York, UK: York Publishing Services.

Carayon, P. (1993). A longitudinal test of Karasek's job strain model among office workers. *Work & Stress, 7*, 299–314.

Carayon, P., Yang, C. L., & Lee, S. Y. (1995). Examining the relationship between job design and worker strain over time in a sample of office workers. *Ergonomics, 38*, 1199–1211.

Clay, R. A. (1998). Downsizing backfires on corporate America. *American Psychological Association Monitor, 29*, 1–2.

Daft, R. L. (2001). *Organization Theory and Design* (7th ed.). Cincinnati, OH: South-Western.

Dawkins, P., & Littler, G. R. (Eds.). (2001). Downsizing: *Is It Working for Australia?* Melbourne: University of Melbourne, Melbourne Institute of Applied Economic and Social Research.

Dawkins, P., Littler, C. R., Venezuela, M. R., & Jensen, B. (1999). *The Contours of Restructuring and Downsizing in Australia* (Report No. ISBN 0-7340-1467-8). Melbourne: University of Melbourne, Institute of Applied Economic and Social Research.

De Jonge, J., & Schaufeli, W. B. (1998). Job characteristics and employee well-being: A test of Warr's Vitamin Model in health-care workers using structural equation modeling. *Journal of Organizational Behavior, 19*, 387–407.

Dekker, S. W. A., & Schaufeli, W. B. (1995). The effects of job insecurity on psychological health and withdrawal: A longitudinal study. *Australian Psychologist, 30*, 57–63.

De-Witte, H. (1999). Job insecurity and psychological well-being: Review of the literature and exploration of some unresolved issues. *European Journal of Work and Organizational Psychology, 8*, 155–177.

Dunlop, Y. (2001). Low-paid employment in the Australian labour market, 1995–97. In J. Borland, B. Gregory, & P. Sheehan (Eds.), *Work Rich, Work Poor* (pp. 95–118). Melbourne: Victoria University, Centre for Strategic Economic Studies.

Edwards, J. R., & Cooper, C. L. (1990). The person-environment fit approach to stress: Recurring problems and some suggested solutions. *Journal of Organizational Behavior, 11*, 293–307.

Fletcher, B., C., & Jones, F. (1993). A refutation of Karasek's demand-discretion model of occupational stress with a range of dependent measures. *Journal of Organizational Behavior, 14*, 319–330.

Ganster, D. C. (1989). Worker control and well-being: A review of research in the workplace. In S. L. Sauter, J. J. Hurrell, & C. L. Cooper (Eds.), *Job Control and Worker Health* (pp. 3–24). Chichester: Wiley.

Gillespie, N. A., Walsh, M., Winefield, A. H., Dua, J., & Stough, C. (2001). Occupational stress in universities: Staff perceptions of the causes, consequences and moderators of stress. *Work and Stress, 15*, 53–72.

Goleman, D. (1995). *Emotional Intelligence*. New York: Bantam Books.

Gouldner, A. W. (1957). Cosmopolitans and locals. *Administrative Science Quarterly, 2*, 282–292.

Grunberg, L., Moore, S. Y., & Greenberg, E. (2001). Differences in psychological and physical health among layoff survivors: The effects of layoff contact. *Journal of Occupational Health Psychology, 6*, 15–25.

Hitt, M. A., Keats, B. W., Harback, H. F., & Nixon, R. D. (1994). Rightsizing – building and maintaining strategic leadership: A long-term competitiveness. *Organizational Dynamics, 23*, 18–32.

Hoel, H., Cooper, C. L., & Faragher, B. (2001). The experience of bullying in Great Britain: The impact of organizational status. *European Journal of Work and Organizational Psychology, 10*, 443–465.

Hoel, H., Rayner, C., & Cooper, C. L. (1999). Workplace bullying. *International Review of Industrial and Organizational Psychology, 14*, 195–230.

Hurrell, J. J., & McLaney, M. A. (1989). Control, job demands, and job satisfaction. In S. L. Sauter, J. J. Hurrell, & C. L. Cooper (Eds.), *Job Control and Worker Health* (pp. 97–103). Chichester: Wiley.

Illing, D. (2001, May 30). Student jam drives staff into overload. *The Australian.*

Jackson, S., & Schuler, R. (1985). A meta-analysis and conceptual critique of research on role ambiguity and role conflict in work settings. *Organization Behavior and Human Decision Processes, 36*, 16–78.

Karasek, R. A. (1979). Job demands, job decision latitude, and mental strain: Implications for job redesign. *Administrative Science Quarterly, 24*, 285–308.

Karasek, R. A. (2001). Toward a psychosocially healthy work environment: Broader roles for psychologists and sociologists. In N. Schneiderman, M. A. Speers, J. M. Silva, H. Tomes, & J. H. Gentry (Eds.), *Integrating Behavioral and Social Sciences with Public Health* (pp. 267–292). Washington, DC: American Psychological Association.

Karasek, R. A., & Theorell, T. (1990). *Healthy Work*. New York: Basic Books.

Katz, D., & Kahn, R. L. (1978). *The Social Psychology of Organizations* (2nd ed.). New York: John Wiley.

Kompier, M. A. J. (1996). Job design and well-being. In M. J. Schabracq, J. A. M. Winnubst, & C. L. Cooper (Eds.), *Handbook of Work and Health Psychology* (pp. 349–368). New York: John Wiley.

Landsbergis, P. A. (1988). Occupational stress among health care workers: A test of the demands-control model. *Journal of Organizational Behavior, 9*, 217–239.

Lubinski, D., & Humphreys, L. G. (1990). Assessing spurious 'moderator effects': Illustrated substantively with the hypothesized ('synergistic') relation between spatial and mathematical ability. *Psychological Bulletin, 107*, 385–393.

Maslach, C., & Leiter, M. P. (1997). *The Truth about Burnout: How Organizations Cause Personal Stress and What to Do about It.* San Francisco: Jossey-Bass Publishers.

Mikkelsen, E. G., & Einarsen, S. (2002). Basic assumptions and symptoms of post-traumatic stress among victims of bullying at work. *European Journal of Organizational Psychology, 11*, 87–111.

Morris, A. J., & Feldman, D. C. (1996). The dimensions, antecedents, and consequences of emotional labor. *Academy of Management Review, 21*, 986–1010.

Narayanan, L., Menon, S., & Spector, P. (1999). Stress in the workplace: A comparison of gender and occupations. *Journal of Organizational Behavior, 20*, 63–74.

National Institute for Occupational Safety and Health. (2002a). *Violence. Occupational Hazards in Hospitals* (No. 2002-110). Cincinnati, OH: NIOSH.

National Institute for Occupational Safety and Health. (2002b). *The Changing Organization of Work and Safety and Health of Working People: Knowledge Gaps and Research Directions* (No. 2002-116). Cincinnati, OH: NIOSH.

O'Driscoll, M. P., & Beehr, T. (2000). Moderating effects of perceived control and need for clarity on the relationship between role stressors and employee affective reactions. *Journal of Social Psychology, 140*, 151–159.

Offermann, L. R., & Malamut, A. B. (2002). When leaders harass: The impact of target perceptions of organizational leadership and climate on harassment reporting and outcomes. *Journal of Applied Psychology, 87*, 885–893.

O'Neill, P. B. (2002). *Validation and cross-validation of a new measure of job security.* Unpublished master's thesis, Curtin University of Technology, Perth, Western Australia, Australia.

Parker, P. A., & Kulik, J. A. (1995). Burnout, self and supervisor related job performance, and absenteeism among nurses. *Journal of Behavioral Medicine, 18*, 581–599.

Parker, S. K., Chmiel, N., & Wall, T. D. (1997). Work characteristics and employee well-being within a context of strategic downsizing. *Journal of Occupational Health Psychology, 2*, 289–303.

Parkes, K. R., Mendham, C. A., & von Rabenau, C. (1994). Social support and the demand-discretion model of job stress: Tests of additive and interactive effects in two samples. *Journal of Vocational Behavior, 22*, 136–147.

Pocock, B. (2002). *The Effects of Long Hours on Family and Community Life.* Adelaide: Adelaide University, Centre for Labour Research.

Probst, T. M. (2002). The impact of job insecurity on employee work attitudes, job adaptation, and organizational withdrawal behaviors. In J. M. Brett, & F. Drasgow (Eds.), *The Psychology of Work: Theoretically Based Empirical Research* (pp. 141–168). Mahwah, NJ: Lawrence Erlbaum Associates.

Reynolds, J. (2001, August). *Layoffs, downsizing, and job insecurity in times of economic prosperity.* Paper presented at the 2001 Annual Meeting of the American Sociological Association, Anaheim, CA.

Robinson, S. L., & Rousseau, D. M. (1994). Violating the psychological contract: Not the exception but the norm. *Journal of Organizational Behavior, 15*, 245–259.

Rosa, R. R. (1995). Extended work shifts and excessive fatigue. *Journal of Sleep Research,* *4,* 51–56.

Rosenblatt, Z., & Ruvio, A. (1996). A test of a multidimensional model of job insecurity: The case of Israeli teachers. *Journal of Organizational Behavior, 17,* 587–605.

Rothschild, J., & Miethe, T. D. (1999). Whistle-blower disclosures and management retaliations: The battle to control information about organization corruption. *Work & Occupations, 26,* 107–128.

Salin, D. (2001). Prevalence and forms of bullying among business professionals. A comparison of two different strategies for measuring bullying. *European Journal of Work and Organizational Psychology, 10,* 425–441.

Salovey, P., & Mayer, J. D. (1990). Emotional intelligence. *Imagination, Cognition, & Personality, 9,* 185–211.

Sauter, S. L., & Hurrell, J. J. (1999). Occupational health psychology: Origins, content, and direction. *Professional Psychology: Research & Practice, 30*(2), 17–122.

Schaubroeck, J., & Jones, J. R. (2000). Antecedents and workplace emotional labor dimensions and moderators of their effects on physical symptoms. *Journal of Organizational Behavior, 21,* 163–183.

Siegrist, J., & Klein, D. (1990). Occupational stress and cardiovascular reactivity in blue collar workers. *Work & Stress, 4,* 295–304.

Sparks, K., Cooper, G., Fried, Y., & Shirom, A. (1997). The effects of hours of work on health: A meta-analytic review. *Journal of Occupational and Organizational Psychology, 70,* 391–408.

Spector, P. E. (1987). Method variance as an artifact in self reported affect and self perceptions at work: Myth or significant problem? *Journal of Applied Psychology, 72,* 438–443.

Sverke, M., & Hellgren, J. (2002). The nature of job insecurity: Understanding employment uncertainty on the brink of a new millennium. *Applied Psychology: An International Review, 51,* 23–42.

Swedish Work Environment Authority. (n.d.). *The state of the working environment.* Retrieved January 13, 2003, from http://www.av.se/english/legislation/chapter2.shtm

Terry, D. J., Nielsen, M., & Perchard, L. (1993). Effects of work stress on psychological well-being and job satisfaction: The stress-buffering role of social support. *Australian Journal of Psychology, 45,* 168–175.

Warr, P. B. (1987). *Work, Unemployment, and Mental Health.* Oxford: Oxford University Press.

Warr, P. B. (1990). Decision latitude, job demands, and employee well being. *Work & Stress, 4,* 285–294.

Warr, P. B. (1994). A conceptual framework for the study of work and mental health. *Work & Stress, 8,* 84–97.

Warr, P. B. (1999). Well-being and the workplace. In D. Kaheman, E. Diener, & N. Schwarz (Eds.), *Well-being: The Foundation of Hedonic Psychology* (pp. 392–412). New York: Russell Sage Foundation.

Wharton, A. S., & Erickson, R. J. (1993). Managing emotions on the job and home: Understanding the consequences of multiple emotional roles. *Academy of Management Review, 18,* 457–486.

WorkSafe (1999). *Code of Practice. Workplace Violence.* Perth, WA: WorkSafe Western Australian Commission.

World Data (1989). *1989 Book of the Year. Encyclopaedia Britannica.* Chicago: Encyclopaedia Britannica.

World Data (1991). *1991 Book of the Year. Encyclopaedia Britannica.* Chicago: Encyclopaedia Britannica.

World Data (2001). *2001 Book of the Year. Encyclopaedia Britannica.* Chicago: Encyclopaedia Britannica.

Worrall, L., & Cooper, C. L. (1998). *Quality of Working Life: 1998 Survey of Managers' Changing Experiences.* London: Institute of Management.

Yang, C. L., & Carayon, P. (1995). Effect of job demands and social support on worker stress: A study of VDT users. *Behavior and Information Technology, 14,* 32–40.

Zapf, D., Seifert, C., Schmutte, B., Mertini, H., & Holz, M. (2001). Emotion work and job stressors and their effects on burnout. *Psychology and Health, 16,* 527–545.

Chapter 12

IDENTIFYING AND MANAGING TRAUMATIC RISK FACTORS EMANATING FROM THE FAMILY–WORK INTERFACE

Jane Shakespeare-Finch and Kathryn Gow

INTRODUCTION

The risk of experiencing traumatic stress is not confined to any particular individual or context. Traumatic events occurring within family systems have the capacity to exert influence on many areas of an individual's life. This chapter identifies traumatic stress risk factors in the family domain and discusses variables that may moderate between the experience and posttrauma outcomes. The discussion is centered within an emergency services context (including police, fire, ambulance, and military services) and presents ways in which an organization can be proactive in aiding an employee to successfully deal with the repercussions of traumatic events experienced within the family system.

Initially, models of the work–family relationship are reviewed. Risk factors are then identified, as are variables postulated to moderate the relationship between work and family domains. Lastly, suggestions for applying this knowledge to preventative risk management strategies are discussed together with the possibility of their being used to facilitate positive posttrauma outcomes (i.e., resilience and posttraumatic growth).

WORK–FAMILY INTERFACE MODELS

In 1990, Lambert provided a comprehensive review of models that aimed to explain the relationship between work and family from an individual's perspective: spillover, compensation, and segmentation. The crossover model, where stress or trauma experienced in the work domain by one partner affects the other partner in a domestic setting, is also relevant here (Bolger, De Longis, Kessler, & Wetherton, 1989; Westman 2001; Westman & Etzion, 1995). As the focus here is more on the movement of traumatic risk from family to work, the crossover model is not elaborated any further. However, this is not to imply that fallout generated from a traumatic experience in the family environment cannot cross over to work, for instance to an employee's partner or colleagues. In this section, we briefly review the major family–work interface models, including the most recent theoretical addition: Border Theory (Campbell Clark, 2000).

Segmentation

Segmentation suggests that events experienced in one domain are largely unrelated to those in another (Lambert, 1990). For example, a trauma in the home environment, such as the serious illness of a family member, does not affect an individual in the workplace because the two domains are cognitively and physically separate (Staines, 1980). Therefore, the contention is that individuals effectively compartmentalize their affect so that one domain is not contaminated by experiences in others. Compartmentalizing issues relating to work and home is a positive coping strategy, whereas, as explained more fully later, dissociation can be a negative and dysfunctional coping strategy. This model is particularly applicable to men who are reputed to have more rigid boundaries than women (Barnett & Marshall, 1992).

Compensation

Compensation describes how changes in one domain relate to changes in others. For example if an employee is dissatisfied with family life, effort and energy are channeled disproportionately into work life. That is, focusing more on the work domain in which the unsatisfying variable is absent compensates for the perceived lack of satisfaction or happiness in the family domain (Lambert, 1990; Sumer & Knight, 2001). This perspective may be related to maladaptive coping strategies in that the employee is avoiding issues in the family system. Furthermore, concentrating all of one's energies on the work domain may lead to burnout and chronic fatigue. Adaptive coping is discussed in more detail later.

Spillover

The spillover model intimates that occurrences in one domain spill over to the other domain (Lambert, 1990; Staines, 1980). Hence, a serious illness within the family can affect the functioning of an employee at work. The spillover model was traditionally conceptualized within a deprivation paradigm and focuses on the negative impact that an event in one domain may have on the other. However, positive spillover has also been identified and is gaining increasing research attention (Grzywacz, Almeida, & McDonald, 2002; Sumer & Knight, 2001; Westman, 2001). That is, a good mood gained via the pleasure of a family wedding, for example, is hypothesized to carry through into the work domain. Over all, research lends the most support to the spillover model, and it is therefore the more prominent model used in current research (Bray, Camlin, Fairbank, Dunteman, & Wheeless, 2001; Grzywacz et al., 2002; Westman, 2001).

Border Theory

Since Lambert's (1990) review, little has changed in terms of explanatory models, with the exception of Campbell Clark's (2000) development of border theory. Border theory conceptualizes that we have borders of various strengths surrounding the family domain and the work domain (and many other domains), and that each day we negotiate the crossing of these borders. Successful negotiation is attributed to factors such as the strength of borders, their permeability, similarities or congruence between domains, and communication (Campbell Clark, 2000). For example, if domains are similar (e.g., caring and responsibility are highly valued in both domains), then weak borders will aid in balancing work and family life. Conversely, when family and work domains are dissimilar (e.g., high value placed on productivity at work versus high value on relaxation at home), the balance between domains is achieved with strong borders.

It can, therefore, be construed that notions of spillover and segmentation are inherent in border theory. Thus, although work–family interface models have been viewed as competing hypotheses (Staines, 1980), it is likely that aspects of each model are present to varying degrees. Border theory may go some way toward addressing the reported inadequacies (Lambert, 1990; Westman, 2001) of previous models in terms of capturing a more complete picture of family and work processes.

As mentioned earlier, the "spillover" of experiences from one domain to another may be negative or positive. Positive experiences within the family domain may have a positive effect on the individual in the work domain (Grzywacz et al., 2002). It is also contended that positive spillover is distinctly different from negative spillover; that is, positive spillover is not simply the absence of stress and/or trauma (Grzywacz, 2000; Westman, 2001). For example, Grzywacz (2000) claims that while less negative spillover is associated with better health outcomes, positive spillover is also related to better health outcomes, independently of that associated with lower levels of negative spillover.

However, most research undertaken in emergency services or military contexts has reported on risk factors that arise in the workplace, rather than in the family, and their potentially negative effects on the family (Pisarski, Bohle, & Callan, 2002; Shakespeare-Finch, Smith, & Obst, 2002; Toch, 2001; Yael, 2002). The following section highlights some of the stress and traumatic stress risk factors that originate from the family system.

FAMILY-RELATED RISK FACTORS

A small body of research has investigated how family stress may influence work life, and a still smaller body of work has highlighted family-related trauma and the influences that it may have on the individual in the workplace. When the individual occupies a position in which the potential for exposure to trauma is relatively high, as in the case of emergency services work, family-related traumatic events may be exacerbated even further. These issues are discussed in more depth later. In this section, we highlight some recent research on family-related factors which may create stress and, moreover, traumatic events in the family domain which may create traumatic stress.

Family-related Stress Risks

Bray et al. (2001) conducted a large study of military personnel ($n =$ 16,193). They examined relationships between work-related, family-related, finance-related, and health-related stress, coping style, substance use, and symptoms of depression, in terms of their relationship with levels of job functioning. They found that both males and females were twice as likely to report work-related stress than family-related stress. Furthermore, family-related stress, maladaptive coping styles, and substance abuse significantly increased the probability of lower levels of job functioning in male personnel but were not significant in the female sample. Similarly, conflicts in military or family domains, the birth of a child, and being away from home were not significantly related to the capacity of females to function at work, but did affect levels of job functioning in males. The researchers suggested that males in the military were less able to manage family-related stressors than females in the military and that this phenomenon may reflect a higher level of skill in females in balancing the demands of both domains (Bray et al., 2001).

Another study that examined family-related stressors and their impact on workplace functioning concluded that fathers who are involved in the primary needs of children (e.g., child-care arrangements, sporting commitments) were most likely to experience a spillover effect (Berry & Rao, 1997). Work–family conflict, such as changes in spousal work schedules and family conflict including calls at work regarding family conflict, was also found to have a negative impact on the work of individuals. Berry and Rao (1997) believe that modern management still regards the family as a woman's domain, and therefore these manifestations of family stress in the workplace may reflect sex-role perspectives. Bray et al. (2001) indicated that the stereotypes associated with sex roles have effected levels of job functioning in the American military.

Although research may indicate that males involved in primary care of children are finding the family and work balancing act more difficult than females, the negatively perceived spillover from family to work attributed to the challenges of balancing work and family life is not peculiar to males. Mothers of young children, in particular, have been found to experience greater levels of spillover from family to work than women without young children (Crouter, 1984), as has being a parent per se (Grzywacz et al., 2002). Indeed, Barnett (1994) found that gender was not a significant issue in the equation, but that marital and parental roles were.

Family-related Traumatic Stress Risks

Personal losses such as a death, divorce, or serious illness, can have a significant impact on an individual worker's capacity to fulfill his or her work-role responsibilities effectively. These factors tend to transcend some of the factors, for example gender differences, that moderate non-traumatic stress risks. Individuals who endure the death of a child, spouse, or significant other, serious illness, separation or divorce may demonstrate difficulties in adjusting to the family-based trauma regardless of gender (Beehr, Johnson, & Nieva, 1995; Bray et al., 2001; Grzywacz et al., 2002).

Other kinds of traumatic risk factors occur in families, such as domestic violence, sexual assault, and witnessing serious injury, and these factors increase the risk of posttraumatic stress disorder (PTSD) (Kessler, Sonnega, Bromet, Hughes, & Nelson, 1995). Similarly, alcohol abuse and suicidal ideation have been identified as a risk for family-to-work spillover (Beehr et al., 1995).

Examining the experience of nonwork trauma and its relationship to work performance and stress in 106 child welfare workers, Digiulio (1995) found that 85% of the participating employees had experienced a personal loss during their current employment. In this research, the workplace was seen as a primary source for facilitating coping mechanisms and, hence, providing an avenue for successfully dealing with nonwork trauma. The identified moderating variables and others are examined in more detail below.

From this brief review, it is evident that risks that emanate from the family system have the potential to effect an individual's level of functioning in the workplace. While factors such as failing child-care arrangements, child illness, quality of marital or parental relationships, or unexpected spousal work schedule changes may create stress for an employee, the death or serious illness of a significant other, divorce, abuse, and several other factors within the family domain can create traumatic stress and significantly alter a worker's capacity to function (Berry & Rao, 1997; Bray et al., 2001; Digiulio, 1995; Grzywacz et al., 2002; Westman, 2001). However, research also demonstrates a capacity for factors such as coping strategies and individual difference variables to moderate or mitigate the relationship between family stress and/or trauma and work performance (Beehr et al., 1995; Burke, 1998; Sumer & Knight, 2001).

MODERATING FACTORS

Individual Difference Variables

People react to traumatic events in various ways. These differences can be partly accounted for by inconsistencies in individual difference variables such as extraversion, openness to experience, optimism, humor, hope, agreeableness, and emotional stability (Berry & Rao, 1997; Moran & Masum, 1997; Shakespeare-Finch, 2003; Tedeschi, Park, & Calhoun, 1998). A sense of control has been associated with levels of resilience in Israeli military personnel (Westman & Etzion, 1995). Kendall, Murphy, O'Neill, and Bursnall (2000) remind us that people differ with regard to what they consider to be stressful. Other issues such as locus of control, thinking patterns (negative or positive), hardiness, coping style, and lack of personal or environmental resources are as important as family–work conflicts.

Recently, notions of both positive and negative spillover of stress from family to work have been linked to attachment styles (Sumer & Knight, 2001). That is, individuals with a preoccupied attachment style experience higher levels of negative spillover from family to work than those with a secure or dismissive attachment style. Reasons for this may be similar to those pertinent to the neurotic individual. People with preoccupied attachment styles and those with higher levels of neuroticism are apparently preoccupied with their own negative feelings and display a tendency to experience negative affect (Sumer & Knight, 2001; Watson & Hubbard, 1996).

Coping Strategies and Social Support

The quality of the marital relationship and the parental relationship can moderate the relationship between the experience of stress and/or trauma and levels of psychological distress (Burke, 1998; Barnett, 1994), as can coping styles, organizational and social support, and marital status (Grzywacz et al., 2002). Beehr et al. (1995) identified four adaptive coping strategies that were used successfully by police officers and their spouses in dealing with family–work stress contagion. They found that problem-focused coping, emotion-focused coping, religiosity, and individualism accounted for the majority of variances in spousal psychological well-being. Spousal support has been found to moderate between the experience of traumatic events and well-being (Broman, Riba, & Trahan, 1996).

Positive spillover to the work environment can be promoted by family life and the perception that a person's spouse understands work issues (Crouter, 1984). Crouter (1984) also found that having a family was advantageous in the work environment because being a parent and a spouse helps an individual to know how to deal with people and how to empathize and understand their issues.

ORGANIZATIONAL RESPONSES AND RESPONSIBILITIES

Identification of At-risk Employees

Although emergency services organizations can reliably determine that certain of their employees will be regularly exposed to traumas, and even though these traumas may be predictable and sometimes overwhelming even for the most resilient individual, they cannot forecast at what point in time, or at what stage of employment, an individual may be more susceptible to experiencing acute stress disorder (ASD) (Bryant & Harvey, 2000) or developing PTSD (*American Psychiatric Association, Diagnostic and Statistical Manual of Mental Disorders*, 1994).

While the full parameters of an "at-risk" profile have not yet been developed for emergency services workers, certain family factors increase the risk of developing aversive reactions to traumatization. Emergency services senior personnel need to be aware of these factors and to have a knowledge of the personal vulnerability of an officer in order to make informed decisions about who may be at risk of experiencing negative reactions in his or her daily work, including attending traumatic incidents that are a normal part of that work. This knowledge and awareness allow senior personnel to assess what type of assignment may be more likely to trigger ASD (and lead on to PTSD) in an employee at certain stages of his or her development or during particularly stressful home/personal life episodes.

Obviously, employers are only responsible for information they have with regard to the officer's home and personal life, and with increasing legislation about privacy, employers may not obtain or request information about the employee's personal life. All of this is very complicated, especially where legal responsibilities are concerned. However, employers need to be able to prove that they have done all within their power with respect to duty of care for their employees who face traumatic events as part of their everyday working life or within the span of their working life. This care extends to understanding the two-way spillover effects between work and home in their human resource policies, selection and induction procedures, staff training, management development, and critical incident protocols.

Triggers for Traumatic Stress

Are traumatic reactions likely to happen with no particular workplace critical incident? The answer is yes. Under a combination of certain workplace conditions of unpredictable, demanding, ongoing changes, higher levels of interpersonal demands and stress, low social support, and a punitive supervision/management style, officers subject to conflicting demands between work and home life, especially those who are under high-level pressure at home because of family demands (the burnout recipe) and unrealistic and sudden, unfair job demands and a relentless pace of work in their employ (burnout and chronic fatigue recipes), are candidates for traumatic stress and in some cases PTSD.

Workplaces of the 21st century have an obligation not to add unfairly to the burden of unmitigated stress and strain on individuals in the workplace. Some work-related stressors outlined by the European Commission (2002) on Health and Safety at work include (1) work overload and underload; (2) lack of support; (3) lack of appreciation or reward; (4) lack of influence/decision latitude; (5) exposure to violence or threat of violence; (6) discrimination and bullying; (7) mistakes causing high costs or risking other people's lives or health; (8) risk of losing one's job; and (9) discrepancy between responsibility and rights. However, with respect to rehabilitation (Kendall et al., 2000), it is unlikely that the workplace will have changed on their return to the workplace, and the stress factors that precipitated the original reaction will remain.

While initially emphasizing the family–work interface, the spillover from workplace to home can be great. When police officers retreat from communicating with their families because they cannot bear to talk about the horrific murder of a child, the senseless bashing of an old woman, or the short-sightedness and corruption of the sociopolitical systems they encounter, the organization needs to recognize the circularity of the problems that appear to have originated from the family but in fact are based in the workplace.

People who have suffered personal trauma previously or who have accumulated trauma responses over several years and those who are currently enduring a trauma are believed to be more vulnerable to workplace trauma. The term "sleeper effect" is of relevance here. It appears in those individuals who apparently show no long-term effects from a trauma until they encounter a trauma within a thematically related area (Greenwald, 2002). Greenwald (2002) conjectures that at some time in the future, when whatever mechanisms that are containing the emotional reactions become overwhelmed, problems emerge. Sometimes people are unaware of the potency of past traumas until some recent event strikes them (Burge, 2002). This does not necessarily mean that they would abreact or become traumatized at work if there were not a workplace critical incident of a serious traumatic kind.

For example, an ambulance officer may cope well with attending to seriously injured road accident victims, both adults and children, for many years; however, if he attends the accident of a five-year-old boy who reminds him in some way of his own five-year-old son and the victim dies, he may well become seriously disturbed and need counseling. This scenario is more likely, however, when he has already lost a five-year-old son and he then attends such a scene. If, in a more serious vein, he has not processed emotionally and ontologically the car accident death of his own son, who was a little boy at the time, and then sees this small boy in front of him, bloodied and broken, he may well abreact, become seriously upset, and suffer from acute posttrauma reactions.

Thus dissociation as a defense from past trauma is not a healthy reaction for those who constantly have to deal with trauma. Post (1992, in Michalski, 1999) notes that "victims of traumatic stressors usually employ psychological defenses to protect themselves from further stimulation" (p. 46); however, this barrier may stop individuals from accepting help, and over time the barrier may become more resistant to penetration. Consequently, Post recommends that posttrauma interventions be conducted early.

Seriously dissociated persons need to be taken out of the line of duty. They are a danger to themselves and others. While in the stress mode, if an officer is in denial or is dissociated from a personal/family trauma and has remained so since the trauma, and if there is evidence of depersonalization (a sense of not being connected to the body or self) together with other signs of an acute or chronic traumatic stress reaction (see American Psychiatric Association, DSM-IV, 1994), the officer may make serious errors of judgment. However, it is important that no attempt be made to break through the person's defense mechanisms, which are a psychological safety mechanism. We cannot stress strongly enough that the person should be dealt with by an appropriately trained licensed health professional of his or her own choice.

A moderate percentage of those who measure highly on ASD (see American Psychiatric Association, DSM-IV, 1994) do develop PTSD. Regardless of where the trauma initiated and the timeline in which the critical incident occurred, employers have a responsibility to assess people who show signs of ASD and then to send them to specialist counseling so that they can avoid developing full-blown symptoms of PTSD. It is also important to note that the percentage of people who go on to develop PTSD is much lower than is popularly believed in the general community.

Speigel (2002) believes that a prior history of trauma and PTSD increases the risk of experiencing traumatic stress. He also says that being in a dissociated state means that the person is in double jeopardy. A person is more likely to be victimized or injured again when in a vulnerable state because he has not cognitively dealt with, emotionally processed, and subsequently integrated the traumatic experience into his life. It is this taxing of certain intellectual faculties to "keep a lid on" the traumatic memories that compounds further problems at work, because that part of the mind which is generally alert – a necessary state for effective emergency services workers – is preoccupied and not fully present on the job.

Assisting Employees At-risk for Traumatic Stress

If an employee in a vulnerable state refuses counseling, a psychologist, employee assistance counselor, or a health and safety officer may be called upon to assess his or her current functioning using an appropriate assessment tool which is interpreted by an appropriately licensed health professional. Employees may be asked to sign a form saying that

they will not hold the organization legally responsible for traumatic reactions to the critical incident. Hence we enter the arena of ethics and
moral principles with respect to duty of care versus the right of privacy
of the individual.

Having new recruits sign a risk waiver for the development of PTSD
or ASD may help in some way to clarify what belongs in the area of
corporate responsibility and what remains in the area of personal responsibility. However, this waiver would not alleviate the onus of duty
of care of the organization should a field officer be called to assist in
some event as unpredictable and momentous as the New York Twin
Towers' incident on September 11, 2001.

Earlier we discussed differences between positive compartmentaliza-
tion and negative dissociation strategies. The distinction between functional and dysfunctional dissociation is too complex and not researched
widely enough to be included here, except to acknowledge that certain
individuals survive trauma well and go on to nonreactive lives simply
because they actually did fully dissociate from the trauma and have no
memory of it whatsoever. That is, they have so successfully not registered the trauma that it does not lay down a neurological pathway in
the memory banks. Hence, it cannot be reactivated.

Thus, simply interviewing people to ascertain their vulnerability in
these matters and assessing them for dissociation tendencies or dissociative abilities will not tell us whether they are likely to abreact badly
in the future. Proper and professional assessment of those who enter the
services could include assessment of factors such as trauma history, dissociative tendencies, coping styles, and personality. However, such
action is not sufficient to avoid committing a Type I error (recruiting
someone who may be at risk of being highly vulnerable to the normal
demands and stresses of the job) or a Type II error (rejecting someone
who may be a first-class and highly capable and resilient officer) and
can lead to charges of discrimination and invasion of privacy.

Recruitment drives and information should contain risk statements
about personal/family trauma and cumulative trauma and the need for
employees to take responsibility for self-care and seeking of counseling
or supervision should the need arise in the course of their duties.
However, new recruits may not like revealing personal information
about personal or family traumas and, if they are forced to do so, may
actually be retraumatized by such insensitivity. Most people do not wish
to revisit traumas if they can avoid doing so.

If the development of PTSD is correlated with the dosage of traumatic exposure, "traumatic events may act as precipitants, the response to which is determined by individual vulnerabilities" (Regehr, Hemsworth, & Hill, 2001, p. 1). These vulnerabilities include biological determinants, cumulative life stressors, previous mental health problems, and a family history of mental illness. There are many factors that may combine and interact with work-related stress to increase the risk of producing or exacerbating PTSD; among those factors of relevance here to emergency services workers are military combat; war and terrorism; random acts of violence in public places, at work, and at school; being an emergency services worker; and being a professional firefighter (Lynn, 2002).

Social Support for Employees under Stress

External factors – social supports and the recovery environment – influence people's responses to such events, and their attachment capacity may interact with social support as a positive factor for an individual (Regehr et al., 2001). This is where social support in the form of a "buddy" is critical. Irrespective of the emergency profession to which individuals are affiliated, their buddies are very important to them. It is their buddies who help to keep them sane and safely grounded in the midst of chaos. The buddy system should be encouraged for mental health stabilizing as long as the buddies are sufficiently sensible to know when to refer to an expert counselor and when to call for emergency help.

We also know that the death of a close buddy will seriously undermine the surviving officer's sense of safety and security. Indeed, while buddies form the major "stuff" of social support for people under constant attack, it is the death of those buddies that makes officers highly vulnerable to "tipping over" the edge. Thus it might be conjectured that those with high affiliation needs are more in danger of developing PTSD than those with low affiliation needs. However, to date, no research has been done on this particular topic to verify such a hypothesis.

Other factors that may impede the return to work include family adjustments to a stress claim, secondary gain, or the maintenance of a sick relative role (Kendall et al., 2000). Nevertheless, on a quite different note, Burge (2002) believes that people come back to work much stronger and with better coping resources after having leave and working through the traumas (Tedeschi, Park, & Calhoun, 1998; Shakespeare-Finch, 2003). Because psychological trauma may be new territory for risk management

(Schneider, 2002), it is often difficult to measure the impact of a critical incident in terms of absenteeism and whether or not those who remain on the job are still fully functioning.

The Need for Organizational Responses: Protocols and Procedures

One reason why critical incident stress debriefing (CISD) may not work effectively (Wessely, Rose, & Bisson, 1998) is that it may not be carried out correctly, in a professionally sensitive way or with the right people. CISD techniques have been nominated (Speigel, 2002) for re-traumatizing people who are suffering from traumatic stress reactions. This does not mean that conducted sensibly and with the right staff in attendance at the right time for the appropriate critical incident, CISD will be detrimental. Nevertheless, staff should have a choice of attending an individual or a group debriefing, and, should they decline, they should not be forced to do so. Perhaps they can simply sign a statement that is was their choice not to attend. From another viewpoint, avoidance or avoidant behavior (if this definitely is the case) is a clear sign that they may need to talk to someone or take time off from work so that their concentration on the job is not impaired and they do not pose a possible danger to themselves or others.

It is not sufficient for health and safety officers alone to be trained in these protocols – all managers and supervisors must be familiar with procedure in the event of a code red. Readers may shrug off the need for emergency services staff to go through this since their core business is full of emergencies. However, some organizations that are set up to help people are not necessarily good at looking after their staff; it is as if the boards and managers expect staff to work under difficult and self-sacrificing conditions without nurturance and care. Because the mission of the organizations is to save lives, or to offer an effective service to the public in emergencies, executives maintain that people who apply to work for such organizations should know this and not expect to be "molly-coddled."

However, employees can have serious reactions to work traumas (e.g., the incident of a staff member committing suicide). Debriefing is important as suicide is a highly traumatic and ontologically threatening act, and it can be contagious, even among highly trained professionals. A lack of alertness is dangerous not only to the self, but to other employees, customers, and the public at large. In order to assess a detached state of mind, simple nonverbal checks and an assessment of speech intonation patterns can be carried out before the person arrives from, or leaves for, home. Similarly, such checks should be conducted when an officer is distressed following an unexpected and upsetting phone call at work.

Stress inoculation training (Lynn, 2002), which is used to help employees deal with stress on the job, emphasizes the three phases of education, skill building, and application. According to Kendall et al. (2000), individual course strategies have a higher profile allowing organizations to be seen to be doing something. These programs tend to include cognitive appraisal, relaxation training, exercise and nutrition, coping skill training or communication, and they may demonstrate short-term efficacy. However, such programs do not address the climatic and cultural sources of work stress (Dollard, 1996, in Kendall et al., 2000), which is really what the organization is culpable for. As Schurman and Israel (1995, in Kendall et al., 2000) point out, in the longer term the organization needs to implement fundamental changes to reduce the stress that employees face in the workplace.

Just as family life can enhance work life (Westman, 2001), organizations can help reduce negative spillover from family stress and trauma. For example, prior to deployment for military duty, stress can be reduced if the military helps with the organization of childcare, legal, and financial arrangements, including the drawing up of wills (Bray et al., 2001). Digiulio (1995) advocates that the workplace facilitate coping with a family-related trauma by offering emotional support, giving additional time off to grieve, providing relief from particularly stressful duties, and offering health and insurance benefits as part of employment packages.

CONCLUSION

In summary, the National Health and Medical Research Council's (2002) guidelines on risk management in the workplace include three recommended steps: (1) identification of hazards, (2) assessment of risk associated with the hazards, and (3) risk control. In relation to traumatic stress, the following actions are required: knowing which incidents and situations are likely to produce traumatic stress reactions (the hazards); assessing their effect (positive and negative); and implementing policies, procedures, and protocols to prevent, reduce, minimize, and manage posttraumatic stress risk. According to the report of the European Commission (2002) on health and safety at work to expand on employers' responsibilities in reducing overall the effects of stressors on employees, nine actions are required:

- Be aware of potential hazards.
- Predict what types of critical incidents emanating from both work and home are likely to increase the likelihood of traumatic stress reactions.
- Identify which employees may be more vulnerable.
- Assess the impact of the trauma on the relevant workers.
- Intervene when it is obvious that the individual employee is negatively affected by a workplace or home-based incident or situation.
- Provide support individually and/or in groups as the unique happening dictates.
- Provide or arrange expert counseling, as needed, for officers whose performance may be impaired, leading to the endangerment of themselves or others.
- Assist employees to reintegrate back into the normal workplace duties as sensitively as possible.
- Help the employee understand that these incidents and situations occur in modern work life and that traumatic stress reactions are a normal reaction to overwhelming and unpredictable events.

In general, work and family/home lives are more closely linked than ever before. Employees work longer hours, often take work home, and, because of technological advances, are increasingly likely to telecommute. When potentially traumatic events occur within the family system, as they do for many people at some stage, the workplace can have a significant impact on resolving posttrauma reactions and may aid in the promotion of an employee's posttrauma resilience and growth.

REFERENCES

American Psychiatric Association. (1994). *Diagnostic and Statistical Manual of Mental Disorders* (4th ed.). Washington, DC: APA.

Barnett, R. C. (1994). Home-to-work spillover revisited: A study of full-time employed women in dual-earner couples. *Journal of Marriage and the Family, 56*, 647–656.

Barnett, R. C., & Marshall, N. L. (1992). Men's job and partner roles: Spillover effects and psychological distress. *Sex Roles, 27*, 455–469.

Beehr, T. A., Johnson, L. B., & Nieva, R. (1995). Occupational stress-coping of police and their spouses. *Journal of Organisational Behaviour, 16*(1), 3–25.

Berry, J. O., & Rao, J. M. (1997). Balancing employment and fatherhood—A systems perspective. *Journal of Family Issues, 18*(4), 386–402.

Bolger, N., De Longis, A., Kessler, R., & Wetherton, E. (1989). The contagion of stress across multiple roles. *Journal of Marriage and the Family, 51*, 175–183.

Bray, R. M., Camlin, C. S., Fairbank, J. A., Dunteman, G. H., & Wheeless, S. C. (2001). The effects of stress on job functioning of military men and women. *Armed Forces and Society, 27*(3), 397–417.

Broman, C. L., Riba, M. L. & Trahan, M. R. (1996). Traumatic events and marital well-being. *Journal of Marriage and the Family, 58*, 908–916.

Bryant, R. A., & Harvey, A. G. (2000). *Acute Stress Disorder: A Handbook of Theory Assessment and Treatment.* Washington, DC: American Psychological Association.

Burge, M. (2002). *Traumatic Shock: How to minimise, manage and recover from it.* Retrieved July 15, 2003, from http://www.actt.com.au/ptsd.html

Burke, R. J. (1998). Work and non-work stressors and well-being among police officers: The role of coping. *Anxiety, Stress, & Coping, 11*(4), 345–362.

Campbell Clark, S. (2000). Work/family border theory: A new theory of work/family interface. *Human Relations, 53*(6), 747–770.

Crouter, A. C. (1984). Spillover from family to work: The neglected side of the work-family interface. *Human Relations, 37*(6), 425–442.

Digiulio, J. F. (1995). A more humane workplace-responding to child welfare workers personal losses. *Child Welfare, 74*(4), 877–888.

European Commission. (2002). Guidance on work-related stress: "*Spice of life – or kiss of death?*" Retrieved July 14, 2003, from http://europa.eu.int/comm/employment_social/publications/2002/ke4502361_en.pdf

Greenwald, R. (2002). *Children's mental health care in the 21st Century: Eliminating the trauma burden.* Retrieved September 12, 2002, from http://www.priory.com/greenwald.htm

Grzywacz, J. G. (2000). Work-family spillover can affect health. *Centre for the Advancement of Health News Release.* Retrieved January 23, 2001, from http://www.cfah.org/hbns/newsrelease/workfamily5-2-00.cfm

Grzywacz, J. G., Almeida, D. M., & McDonald, D. A. (2002). Work-family spillover and daily reports of work and family stress in the adult labour force. *Family Relations: Interdisciplinary Journal of Applied Family Studies, 51*(1), 28–36.

Kendall, E., Murphy, P., O'Neill, V., & Bursnall, S. (2000). *Occupational stress: Factors that contribute to its occurrence and effective management.* Retrieved July 14, 2003, from http://www.workcover.wa.gov.au/PDF/Occupational%20Stress.pdf

Kessler, R. C., Sonnega, A., Bromet E., Hughes, M., & Nelson, C. B. (1995). Posttraumatic stress disorder in the National Comorbidity Survey. *Archives of General Psychiatry, 52*, 1048–1060.

Lambert, S. J. (1990). Processes linking work and family: A critical review of the research agenda. *Human Relations, 43*(3), 239–257.

Lynn, L. M. (2002). Updates on the diagnosis and treatment of PTSD with children, adults and the elderly. *Continuing Education Services.* Retrieved September 14, 2002, from http://www.homestudyceu.com

Michalski, J. H. (1999). *Improving Family Services: Linking outcomes and research results with practice.* Retrieved July 16, 2003, from http://www.cprn.com/docs/family/ifs_e.pdf

Moran, C., & Masum, M. (1997). An evaluation of humour in emergency work. *The Australasian Journal of Disaster and Trauma Studies, 3.* Retrieved July 14, 1999, from http://www.massey.ac.nz/%7Etrauma

National Health and Medical Research Council. (2002). *When It's Right in Front of You: Assisting Health Care Workers in Rural and Remote Australia to Manage Episodes of Violence.* Canberra, Australia: NHMRC.

Pisarski, A., Bohle, P., & Callan, V. J. (2002). Extended shifts in ambulance work: Influences on health. *Stress & Health, 18*(3), 119–126.

Regehr, C., Hemsworth, D., & Hill, J. (2001). Individual predictors of posttraumatic distress: A structural equation model. *Canadian Journal of Psychiatry, 46,* 156–161.

Regehr, C., Hill, J., & Glancy, G. D. (2000). Individual predictors of traumatic reactions in firefighters. *The Journal of Nervous and Mental Disease, 188*(6), 333–339.

Schneider, D. (2002). Workplace catastrophes demand a specialized approach. *IntraSpectives: News and views on the disability management industry, 2*(1). Retrieved October 31, 2002, from http://www.intracorp.com/IntracorpHome/intraspectives/d/january/print/

Shakespeare-Finch, J. E. (2003). *Posttraumatic growth in emergency ambulance personnel: The roles of personality and coping.* Unpublished doctoral dissertation, Queensland University of Technology, Brisbane, Australia.

Shakespeare-Finch, J. E., Smith, S. G., & Obst, P. (2002). Trauma, coping and family functioning in emergency service workers. *Work and Stress, 16*(3), 275–282.

Speigel, D. (2002). *The use of hypnosis in treating trauma.* Paper presented at the Society for Clinical and Experimental Hypnosis' 53rd Annual Congress, Boston, MA.

Staines, G. L. (1980). Spillover versus compensation: A review of the literature on the relationship between work and non-work. *Human Relations, 33*(2), 111–129.

Sumer, H. C., & Knight, P. A. (2001). How do people with different attachment styles balance work and family? A personality perspective on work-family linkage. *Journal of Applied Psychology, 86*(4), 653–663.

Tedeschi, R. G., Park, C. L., & Calhoun, L. (Eds.). (1998). *Posttraumatic Growth: Positive Changes in the Aftermath of Crisis.* New Jersey: Lawrence Erlbaum Associates.

Toch, H. (2001). *Stress in Policing.* Washington, DC: American Psychological Association.

Watson, D., & Hubbard, B. (1996). Adaptational style and dispositional structure: Coping in the context of the five-factor model. *Journal of Personality, 64*(4), 737–774.

Wessely, S., Rose, S., & Bisson, J. (1998). A systematic review of brief psychological interventions ("debriefing") for the treatment of immediate trauma related symptoms and the prevention of post traumatic stress disorder (Cochrane Review). *The Cochrane Library, 4.*

Westman, M. (2001). Stress and strain crossover. *Human Relations, 54*(6), 717–751.

Westman, M., & Etzion, D. (1995). Crossover of stress, strain and resources from one spouse to another. *Journal of Organisational Behavior, 16*(2), 169–181.

Yael, D. (2002). *Sharing the Front Line and the Back Hills: International Protectors and Providers: Peacekeepers, Humanitarian Aid Workers and the Media Amidst Crisis.* Amityville, NY: Baywood Publishing.

Chapter 13

TERRORISM AND TRAUMA: THE DIMENSION OF FEAR

John M. Violanti

"Freedom and fear are at war."
George W. Bush

INTRODUCTION

On September 11, 2001, a flood of fear streamed over citizens of the United States, fear brought about by a calculated terrorist attack on their own soil. For the first time, Americans experienced the invasiveness of foreign terror at home. Symbolic landmarks were the chosen targets of these terrorists, and, in the end, the World Trade Center was destroyed and the Pentagon badly damaged. As rescue personnel rushed to help, they too fell victim to fire, explosions, and collapsing buildings. Lipton (2001) reported the demographics of death in *The New York Times:*

- Total dead: estimated 2,825 persons.
- Three times as many men as women died.
- Majority of the dead were between the ages of 35–39.
- Ninety-eight percent were at work in their offices.
- Victims were residents from 25 states.
- Of the victims from New York City, 330 were from Manhattan, 283 from Brooklyn, 242, from Queens, 183 from Staten Island, and 89 from the Bronx.
- The youngest victim was $2\frac{1}{2}$ years old; the eldest 85 years of age.

- Of foreign victims, the United Kingdom had the greatest number with fifty-three.
- All but nine died on the day of the attack.
- Only 986 of the 2,825 victims have been positively identified.

Americans had witnessed a horrible act of terrorism six years earlier in Oklahoma City when 168 people died in the bombing of the Alfred P. Murrah Federal Building. This time it was different; a foreign invader, Al Queda, had infiltrated their lives. Americans had generally believed that the homeland was a safe place – that foreign terrorists only blew up buildings in other countries. There was a realization that safety at home may only be an illusion, never again to be regained. Indeed, the lives of Americans had changed forever.

Acts of terrorism are close to disasters in appearance, but with an important difference. Terrorism is, in the first instance, intentional and has the purpose of intimidation and coercion, as well as inducing a sense of helplessness and confusion among the targeted population. Terrorism has the potential to overwhelm even the most carefully planned disaster response plans, especially when weapons of mass destruction such as biological, chemical, or nuclear weapons are used (Jacobs & Kulkarni, 1999).

TERRORISM AND FEAR

One of the goals of this book is to focus on the qualities of traumatic events which impact traumatic reactions and posttraumatic stress disorder (PTSD) in individuals. This chapter concerns a central quality of terrorism: the propagation of fear among a selected population. Fear has been categorized as a preponderant quality of trauma (American Psychiatric Association, *Diagnostic and Statistical Manual of Mental Disorders*, 1994). Figure 13.1 illustrates a simple model of the terrorism-fear-trauma hypothesis.

The model initially suggests that acts of terrorism purposefully attempt dissemination of fear in targeted populations The terrorists then anticipate that the fear caused by their acts will generalize to the entire population and will endure. Thus, it is posited that, in many cases, the goal of terrorism is more to establish fear to bring about desired political or social change than to simply kill people. The destruction of life and property, however, may be an additional goal of terrorists.

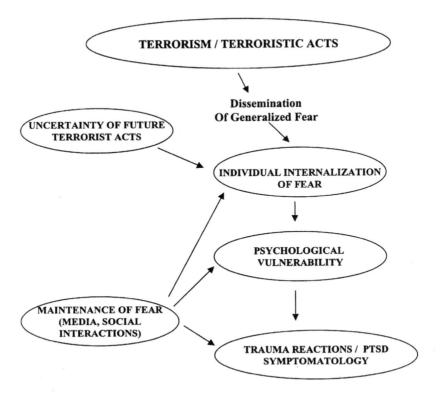

Figure 13-1. Terrorism, fear, and trauma model.

There are many established viewpoints as to how and why terrorism uses fear as a primary motivation for bringing change. In fact, the term "terrorism" itself has been the subject of great debate. There are some who think that terrorism is nothing more than senseless violence, fueled by hatred for another race or religion or group. But most believe that the terrorist acts with conviction; there exists a motivation to change some policy or societal code (White, 1998). There is agreement in most definitions of terrorism, however, that fear is the primary weapon. Rosie (1987), for example, points out that persons frightened into surrender or compliance are the real targets of terrorism. It does not matter if people are killed or injured; what matters is that the target population is frightened:

> The use and/or threat of repeated violence in support of or in opposition to some authority [constitutes terrorism], where violence is applied to induce fear of similar attack in as many non-immediate victims as possible so that those threatened accept the demands of the terrorists (p. 7).

Jenkins (1985) stated that "terrorism is theater"; that terrorist acts are intended to establish fear in an audience in order to influence their behavior and actions. Jenkins offers a simple definition of terrorism as "the use or threatened use of force designed to bring about political change" (p. 8). In Schmid's (1983) syntheses of terrorism definitions, he found that fear was one of the two most commonly appearing elements in conceptualizations of terrorism. He commented that "violent actors" can instill a chronic state of fear by using violence outside the realm of normal behavior. This in turn produces fear in the general audience beyond immediate victims and motivates attitude change in the larger population.

More recently, Cooper (2001) defined terrorism as "the intentional generation of massive fear by human beings for the purpose of securing or maintaining control over other human beings" (p. 883). Implicit in this definition is the use of fear as a method of social control. According to Cooper, any definition of terrorism must consider the central feature of massive fear:

> Creating massive fear in human beings is based on the same principles that have always informed the process: You can kill them, you can mutilate them or otherwise damage their physical or mental integrity, you can deprive them of their liberty, you can damage or destroy their relationships with people and things, you can adversely alter the quality of their lives by affecting their environment or their economic prospects or by imposing onerous burdens on them, or you can achieve your ends by credibly threatening to do all or any of these things. It is not possible to conceive of anything else that might accomplish the goal of creating the massive fear, or terror, that is the heart of terrorism (p. 886).

An emerging problem concerns the advancement of even more horrendous methods to induce fear. *Weapons of mass destruction* (WMD) has become a buzz phrase among counter-terrorist forces, indicating that large numbers of people can be killed or injured with the use of nuclear, chemical, or biological weapons. Even more terrifying is the fact that such weapons can be "weaponized" by rather simple mechanisms. Recent use of the U.S. Postal system to spread anthrax is a primary example. In addition, the terrorist's audience is now more difficult to impress or shock (Cooper, 2001). In the past, the assassination of a dignitary might have sufficed to disrupt a population and cause widespread fear. Today, it takes much more horrendous acts to achieve such results. Al Queda, for example, found it necessary to destroy the World Trade Center and Pentagon to make a political point. Cooper comments:

As in so many other departments of modern life, the audience has become increasingly difficult to shock. Indeed, the terrorist nowadays has to struggle mightily against a kind of ennui affecting those he or she would seek to impress. The audience, with the ever present assistance of television reporting of the contemporaneous, has become sated on a diet of death and destruction. The misery of others is fast losing its ability to horrify or, at least, to horrify for very long. This has made the terrorist's task increasingly difficult: How do you recapture and refocus the jaded attention of such an audience? The possibilities are really quite limited. You can strive to increase the toll in terms of the body count; compared to conventional warfare, deaths resulting from acts of terrorism have been numerically insignificant. the terrorist has to imagine novel, strikingly horrible means for doing the traditional things; and, significantly, the execution must match the imaginings. Clearly, whichever course is chosen, some of the mystery has to be reintroduced. Fear feeds off the unknown (p. 888).

Thus, we come to the conclusion that terrorism is only secondarily aimed at death and destruction. The ultimate goal appears instead to instill fear in a population for purposes of influencing attitudes and behaviors. Fear has its psychological consequences, as we now consider the impact of the terrorist's acts.

PERSONAL VULNERABILITY AND TERRORISM

The risk of exposure to terrorism has taken on new meaning since 9/11. The relationship between terroristic exposure and psychological trauma may be mediated by individual vulnerabilities as they apply to fear. Cooper (2001) commented that the "bad news" about terrorism is that it not only will increase in the future, but also will become more destructive and deadly. The ability of the media to instantaneously bring the horrible details of a terrorist event directly into the home will no doubt increase not only exposure to terror but also personal vulnerability to its impact. There is little chance to avoid the flooding of information resources with news of terroristic acts.

The potential for traumatic stress generally includes vulnerability as a determinant of differences in individual susceptibility to negative life events (Paton, Smith, Violanti, & Eränen, 2000). Blaikie, Cannon, Davis, & Wisner (1994) defined vulnerability as the combination of characteristics of a person or group in terms of their capacity to anticipate, cope with, resist, and recover from hazard impacts that threaten their lives, well-being, and livelihood. Violanti (1990) described how personal vulnerability interacts with traumatic events, commenting that it cannot account for the complex relationship between psychological distress and traumatic events. Many persons so exposed do not suffer psychological consequences, yet others experience extreme reactions. Because of the complex interaction of individual differences, environmental influences, and socialization factors, it is difficult to obtain an individual indicator of vulnerability. The next best available measure would be a vulnerability coefficient, estimated as a constant across a group of individuals. Such coefficients can be statistically applied within and between groups at risk of trauma exposure.

Differences in individual trauma reactions within the literature have heightened awareness of differential vulnerability (Paton, et al., 2000). Scotti, Beach, Northrop, Rode, & Forsyth (1995) identified three categories. The first concerned biological factors and genetically-based predispositions (e.g., heightened autonomic and physiological reactivity) and changes in physiological reactivity as a consequence of prior traumatic exposure. Secondly, historical antecedents such as learning history, experience of child abuse, and pre-existing psychopathology are influential. Finally, psychological factors such as learned avoidance of threat situations, social skills deficits that limit use of social support, hypervigilance of threat-relevant cues, and inadequate problem-solving behavior affect vulnerability. Vulnerability can also be influenced by the person's history of traumatic experience prior to employment (Paton, 1999). Important issues here are the nature, frequency, timing, and extent of resolution of such experiences. Transient factors such as health status, fatigue, and psychological fitness can increase trauma stress vulnerability.

SHATTERED ASSUMPTIONS OF SAFETY

Despite a long-held belief that their home soil was relatively safe from foreign attack, Americans lost this perception of safety after the events of 9/11. Feelings of intense anxiety and helplessness accompany this lost sense of safety and security (Figley, 1985). The fear instilled by terrorism works by breaking down the walls of psychological invulnerability. A new perception of vulnerability manifests itself because of the terrorism exposure, dominated by preoccupation with the fear of recurrence. Once one is victimized, it is relatively easy to see oneself in the role again; the experience is now "available," and one sees oneself as "representative" of those victimized (Kahneman & Tversky, 1973).

That 9/11 was a human-induced act made it particularly distressing for Americans and compounded the loss of perceived safety and security. The accuracy of this statement is is reflected in the huge decrease in airline use and travel immediately following the attack. Myers (2001) stated that the terrorists made progress in their fear war by diverting our anxieties from big risks toward smaller risks. Thus, the American illusion of invulnerability was shattered at the macro- and at the everyday-existence micro-levels. To Americans, the world is now a threatening place – terrorism has come home and is no longer deniable.

Consequently, the American nation sees itself as seriously challenged. The assumptions that formerly enabled this nation to function effectively no longer serve as guides for behavior (Janoff-Bulman & Freize, 1983). Daw (2001) commented that Americans must explore a new way of being. Feelings of terrorism vulnerability must be kept within bounds in order that people can continue to function normally. Samuel Karson (quoted in Murray, 2001), an FAA psychologist, commented that feelings of vulnerability can be assuaged if we deal with our weakness of not knowing the intention of our enemies. Massive information is thus needed on the terrorists, their culture, language, and psychology. Zimbardo (2001) stated that the fear generated by terrorism undercuts our sense of trust, stability, and confidence in our personal world. Fear becomes anxiety when it generalizes to become a more pervasive feeling of personal vulnerability.

POSTTRAUMATIC STRESS, FEAR, AND TERRORISM

Posttraumatic stress reactions can result from a variety of exposures. Among the context of these events, *fear* is considered an important factor is the etiology of PTSD. The DSM-IV (American Psychiatric Association, 1994) lists fear among its "*Criteria A*" for PTSD. Brewin, Andrews, and Rose (2000) conducted a longitudinal analysis of fear to determine its validity. They found that this PTSD criterion is justified. Sixty-one percent of those diagnosed with PTSD reported "intense" trauma-related emotions of fear at six months postevent.

Feelings of vulnerability and fear that result from terrorist acts may be persistent and thus have the potential to pose a much higher risk for

PTSD than most other disasters, which are temporary in nature. In addition, unlike in natural disasters, the fear and feelings of vulnerability generated by terrorism have the capability to spread to general as well as local populations.

In regard to the 9/11 attacks on the World Trade Center and Pentagon, some 100,000 people directly witnessed the event, and millions more witnessed it through the media (Shuster et al., 2001; Yehuda, 2002). The consequent potential for psychological trauma is immense. Shuster et al. (2001) conducted a nationwide study three to five days after the attack to assess the mental health effect of the attack. Their findings indicate that 44% of the nationally representative sample reported that they had at least one of five substantial stress symptoms since the attacks, and 90% reported at least low levels of stress symptoms. Thirty-five percent of children also experienced stress. Shuster et al. (2001) also reported that the World Trade Center attack affected those who were not physically present. This was true for other disasters: the Challenger explosion (Terr, Bloch, Michel, Shi, Reinhardt, & Metayer, 1999), the Gulf War (Cantor, Mares, & Oliver, 1993), and the Oklahoma City bombing (Pfefferbaum, Seale, McDonald, Brandt, Rainwater, Maynard, et al., 2000). The Shuster et al. (2001) study survey indicated that Americans responded to the attacks in various ways:

> Most turned to religion, and also to one another for social support. They checked on the safety of those they cared about, talked about their thoughts and feelings, and participated in activities such as vigils, which can provide a sense of community. They also made donations. Efforts to help people far away, which have been reported after other tragedies, may have been means of coping in the aftermath of the attacks – trying to take constructive action in a time of uncertainty and helplessness. Some people avoided activities, such as watching television, that reminded them of the attacks. Although it has been postulated that avoidance interferes with the emotional processing necessary to recover fully from trauma, the unusual circumstances and continuous coverage of the September 11 attacks may have made avoidance in the short term a healthy response (p. 1511).

A study by Galea, Ahern, Resnick, Kilpatrick, Bucuvalas, Gold, and Vlahov (2002) assessed the psychological sequelae of the 9/11 attacks in New York City. In their representative sample of adults living south of 110th street in Manhattan five to eight weeks after the attack, 7.5% of respondents reported symptoms of PTSD, and 9.7% reported symptoms of depression. These findings suggest that 67,000 persons had

PTSD and 87,000 had depression at the time of the study. They also found that persons directly affected by the New York City attack had higher levels of PTSD than those in more distant sections of Manhattan. Concerning possible protective factors, Galea et al. (2002) reported that low levels of social support were related to both PTSD and depression. This finding is similar to those in other disaster studies (Fullerton, Ursano, Kao, & Bharitya, 1999).

CHEMICAL AND BIOLOGICAL TERRORISM

The threat of bioterrorism is very real. At least seventeen nations are believed to have offensive biological weapons programs (Inglesby, Henderson, Ascher, Eitzen, Friedlander, et al., 1999; Cole, 1996). Iraq has acknowledged producing and weaponizing anthrax (Zilinskas, 1997). The terrorist organization that released sarin in a Tokyo, Japan, subway station (WuDunn, Miller, & Broad, 1998) dispersed aerosols of anthrax and botulism throughout Tokyo on at least eight occasions. The accidental release of anthrax from a military facility in the former Soviet Union resulted in at least 79 cases of anthrax infection and 68 deaths and demonstrated the lethal potential of anthrax (Meselson, Guillemin, & Hugh-Jones, 1994). The World Health Organization (WHO) estimated that casualties following the release of 50 kilograms of anthrax over a dense population of 5 million would be 250,000 (World Health Organization, 1970). The United States Congressional Office of Technology Assessment estimated that between 130,000 and 3 million deaths could follow the release of 100 kilograms of anthrax in the Washington, D.C. area (US Congressional Office of Technology Assessment, 1993).

Weapons of mass destruction (WMD) have great potential for increasing fear and psychological symptomatology among huge segments of a population. The recent anthrax scare in the United States demonstrates how biological terrorism can spread fear through an entire population. Two weeks after the meltdown at the Three Mile Island nuclear plant, 26% of the local population showed a "demoralization." A year and half later, persons in the residential area of the plant reported stress, somatic complaints, and high levels of anxiety (Smith, North, & Price, 1988). After the first missile attack on Israel in the Persian Gulf war, nearly 40% of civilians in the immediate area had somatic symptoms related to chemical exposure, even though there was none (Carmeli,

Liberman, & Mevorach, 1991). In the Tokyo sarin gas subway attack, over 30% reported chemical-related symptoms, but had none. One month after the incident, 32% of those treated reported fear of subways, 29% reported sleep disturbances, and 16% reported flashbacks and depression (DiGiovanni, 1999; Ohbu et al., 1997). In the recent anthrax mail attacks, many reported biological exposure symptoms without actually being exposed to the agent (Center for Disease Control, 2001).

PSYCHOLOGICAL IMPLICATIONS
OF DISASTERS AND SUICIDE

Although PTSD and depression have been the subjects of previous research, less is known about suicide as it relates to disaster events. Studies of the effects of disasters on suicide rates have yielded insufficient information, primarily because they have focused only on suicidal ideation or because they have looked at single disasters with populations too small to allow significant comparisons to be made between predisaster and postdisaster suicide rates (Imamura, 1995; Lew & Wetli, 1996; Warheit, Zimmerman, Khoury, Vega, & Gil, 1996). Given the link between disasters and depression, as well as the link between depression and suicide, it is reasonable to expect a relation between disasters and suicide rates.

Krug et al. (1998) demonstrated that suicide rates increased by 13.8% during the four years after a severe natural disaster. Increased rates were found for both sexes and for all age groups. During the same period, suicide rates in the United States as a whole remained stable.

There are several possible reasons why people may commit suicide after or during a disaster. First, a choice for suicide may occur. For example, during the World Trade Center attack on 9/11, many people jumped from the Trade Center rather than face certain death in the building. Second, victims may suffer many losses due to the disaster: family members, friends, property, and so on (Bolin, 1985; Gerrity & Flynn, 1997). Disasters of the proportions of 9/11 can also lead to loss of place as well. The daily routine is upset; restaurants, facilities, and so on are no longer there.

Feelings of social support and belonging often decline after natural disasters (Kaniasty, Norris, & Murrell, 1995). Disruption of social networks has been associated with mental health problems, including depression and hopelessness (Solomon, 1992). The Krug et al. (1998) study suggests that mental health support is needed after severe disasters, that it should be available for varying periods, and that it should accommodate the needs of various age groups. Prevention could include providing social support and facilitating aid to victims. In addition, disaster-prone areas could be targeted for programs that reduce the conditions that predispose people to commit suicide.

MAINTENANCE OF FEAR: TERRORISM AND THE MEDIA

Terrorism thrives on media exposure since its goal is to spread fear to as large an audience as possible (Schechterman & Slann, 1993). The influence of the media on the attitudes and emotional state of people is a subject of debate (Slone, 2000; Lee, 1990; Curran, Gurevitch, & Woollacott, 1982). Some researchers have hypothesized that media presentation of violence and death brings about emotions of fear among the exposed audience (Slone, 2000).

A point of contention is the uneasy balance between freedom of the press and media control. Kidder (1993) questions whether media reporting is news or propaganda. He terms television as "the stage on which terrorist incidents are played" (p. 130). Ted Koppel, ABC Television's "Nightline" host, made the following comment:

> American television is particularly vulnerable to misuse. We are vulnerable to misuse by our own leaders. We are vulnerable to misuse by our international adversaries. And they obviously include terrorists. The fact that terrorism by definition tends to be dramatic, [and] the fact that by definition it tends to involve acts which are pictorial, makes us even more vulnerable. [But] don't make the mistake of jumping to the conclusion that the immediate impact of that day's visual message is the final impact. The American media . . . operate under what ultimately is our basic assumption in this country, a Jeffersonian notion, that if you allow the public access to all the information, no matter how dramatic or devastating it may be at any given point, ultimately they will reach the proper conclusions (Quoted in Schechterman & Slann, 1993, p. 133).

The question for discussion is the psychological impact of the media reporting of terrorist incidents. Shuster et al. (2001) commented that media exposure to the New York City 9/11 attack was prolonged and detailed and served as a traumatic reminder to all of the day's horrible events. Shuster et al. further reported that 39% of their national sample avoided watching television after the 9/11 event because it reminded them of what happened. Children appeared vulnerable to trauma symptoms if they watched coverage of 9/11 unabated by their parents. A strong positive relationship was found between hours of television watched and reported stress symptoms. Recommendation for restriction of children to media exposure was proposed in this study. Slone's (2000) analysis of exposure to media presentation of terrorist threats among Israelis found an association between such broadcasts and psychological symptomatology. She comments that these findings suggest that media coverage of terrorism is not benign as some would suggest, but has a powerful and potentially damaging impact on the psychological well-being of the public. Schmid and DeGraff (1982) place the blame for the impact of terrorism on the media. These authors conclude that the media, by virtue of their power and influence, should essentially police themselves. They believe the media's task is to operate as effective agents of positive social change, rather than to compete with one another for ratings and audiences.

Freedom of the press is essential in a democratic society. The public has the right to know and understand recent events, especially those that directly impact their everyday life. The media has a difficult balance to maintain in reporting events such as 9/11. On one side is the public's need to know. Citizens must be kept informed of such critical events to help them deal with crises. On the other side, it is very possible that exposure to media coverage can cause psychological discomfort and distress. The responsibility for ethical reporting by the media is necessary, as well as the responsibility of the public to limit their exposure if so warranted. This need to limit exposure is especially true for children (Shuster, et al., 2001).

CONCLUSIONS

"Fears are educated into us, and can, if we wish, be educated out."
Karl A. Menniger

To a great degree, those who perpetrated the 9/11 attack and other terrorists have been successful. Although the have not successfully overthrown governments or substantially destroyed infrastructures, they have instilled fear in populations. That may very well have been their primary goal. Citizens of Israel must walk in fear in public places, never knowing when a suicide bomber might attack. In the United States, an Office of Home Security now exists where none had existed before. Americans have become more vigilant in their observations of foreign-born persons; immigration laws have tightened; and an underlying fear is prevalent among air travelers. Americans no longer have a feeling of safety at home, a feeling they took for granted in the past. The task now is to deal effectively with the psychological impact of terrorism. The following are some suggestions.

Bartone (2001) provides four important recommendations for leaders and supervisors following disasters and terrorist attacks such as 9/11. First, there is an immediate temptation for leaders to gloss over the step of experiencing and reflecting on the loss. The risk here is that they will be perceived by subordinates and community members as insensitive and uncaring. Leaders generate solidarity and healing in their organizations by modeling appropriately sad reactions to tragic losses.

Second, leaders can help community members to make a mental link between the loss and going on with life. Rather than ignore the event, they can call attention to it directly and, at the same time, explain that attending to normal tasks is an appropriate and important response to what has happened.

Third, communication is important. In the aftermath of disasters there are great uncertainty and confusion. Leaders can generate a sense of trust and solidarity in their organizations by frequently sharing what they know and what they do not know. On the other side of the coin, leaders can inadvertently increase the uncertainty and sense of lost moorings by not telling people in their organizations what is going on.

Finally, memorial services are important. In the days and weeks following the tragedy, community memorial and prayer services are an important way for people to come together, recognize the loss, and provide mutual support. Such events also provide a platform for leaders to exercise effective "grief leadership." At memorial services, leaders can demonstrate their own acceptance of the loss, while also helping the community to interpret these tragic events in a way that facilitates renewed cooperative effort.

Calhoun and Tedeschi (2000) offer a positive growth model for intervention into traumatic events such as 9/11. They view trauma as an opportunity for people to grow, suggesting that the struggle with highly challenging circumstances can produce significant positive changes for many persons coping with trauma. Individuals do not simply survive without negative effects; they experience themselves as better than they were before the traumatic event. In work with those exposed to highly traumatic events, a key component of intervention is to assist each person to recover a sense of safety (Herman, 1992). A similar process is also an important consideration for brief, early posttraumatic interventions designed for groups, such as critical incident debriefings. The need for a sense of safety not only applies to any immediate physical threat, but also to the general sense that the posttraumatic intervention itself is "safe" (Calhoun & Tedeschi, 2000).

What philosophical strategies can help terrorism victims deal with feelings of fear? According to DeBecker (1998), too many people walk around in constant fear, their intuition misinformed about what really poses danger. True fear should be temporary in nature and serve only as a survival signal that sounds in the presence of danger. It is the ultimate goal of terrorism to instill terror in people, terror that will be long lasting and serve to control or change the minds of those exposed. To dismantle the emotional impact of fear on psychological well-being, one must consider dismantling hypervigilance. DeBecker (1998) poses two "rules" about fear:

> First, the very fact that you fear something is solid evidence that it is not happening. Fear is a concern of what might happen next. Secondly, what you fear is rarely what you think you fear – it is what you link to fear. If fear is real, it will be linked to the presence of danger, injury, or death (p. 342).

As the war on terrorism continues throughout the world, those on the home front must pledge to continue their lives without fear and disruption. That is the individual's best psychological "weapon" for victory over fear and trauma, and, ultimately, over terrorism.

REFERENCES

American Psychiatric Association. (1994). *Diagnostic and Statistical Manual of Mental Disorders* (4th ed.). Washington, DC: APA.

Bartone, P. T. (2001). *Information paper on leader issues in the aftermath of 11 SEP 2001 terrorist strike at the World Trade Center and the Pentagon.* Internal memorandum presented at the United States Military Academy, West Point, NY.

Blaikie, P., Cannon, T., Davis, I., & Wisner, B. (1994). *At Risk: Natural Hazards, People's Vulnerability and Disaster.* London: Rutledge.

Bolin, R. (1985). Disaster characteristics and psychosocial impacts. In B. J. Sowder (Ed.), *Disasters and Mental Health: Selected Contemporary Perspectives* (pp. 3–28). Washington, DC: US Government Printing Office.

Brewin, C. R., Andrews, B., & Rose, S. (2000). Fear, helplessness, and horror in post-traumatic stress disorder: Investigating DSM-IV criterion A2 in victims of violent crime. *Journal of Traumatic Stress, 13,* 499–509.

Calhoun, L. G., & Tedeschi, R. G. (2000). Early posttraumatic interventions: Facilitating possibilities for growth. In J. M. Violanti, D. Paton, & C. Dunning (Eds.), *Posttraumatic Stress Intervention: Challenges, Issues, and Perspectives* (pp. 135–152). Springfield, IL: Charles C Thomas.

Cantor, J., Mares, M. L., & Oliver, M. B. (1993). Parents and children's emotional reaction to TV coverage of the Gulf war. In B. S. Greenberg, & W. Gantz (Eds.), *Desert Storm and the Mass Media* (pp. 156–178). Cresskill, NJ: Hampton Press.

Carmeli, A., Liberman, N., & Mevorach, L. (1991). Anxiety related somatic reaction during missile attacks. *Israeli Journal of Medical Science, 27,* 677–680.

Center for Disease Control. (2001). Update: Investigation of anthrax associated with intentional exposure and interim public health guidelines. *Morbidity and Mortality Weekly Report, 50,* 889–896.

Cole, L. A. (1996). The specter of biological weapons. *Scientific American, 12,* 60–65.

Cooper, H. H. A. (2001). Terrorism: The problems of definition revisited. *American Behavioral Scientist, 44,* 881–893.

Curran, J. M., Gurevitch, M., & Woollacott, J. (1982). The study of the media: Theoretical approaches. In M. Gurevitch, T. Bennet, J. Curran, & J. Woollacott (Eds.), *Culture, Society and the Media* (pp. 58–73). London: Rutledge.

Daw, J. (2001). Responding to the nation's sadness, anger and fear. *Monitor on Psychology, 32.* Retrieved July 3, 2002 from www.apa.monitor/nov01/

DeBecker, G. (1998). *The Gift of Fear.* New York: Dell.

DiGiovanni, C. (1999). Domestic terrorism with chemical and biological agents: Psychiatric aspects. *American Journal of Psychiatry, 156,* 1500–1505.

Figley, C. R. (1985). *Trauma and Its Wake.* New York: Brunner/Mazel.

Fullerton, C. S., Ursano, R. J., Kao, T. C., & Bharitya, V. R. (1999). Disaster-related bereavement: Acute symptoms and subsequent depression. *Aviation and Space Environmental Medicine, 70,* 902–909.

Galea, S., Ahern, J., Resnick, H., Kilpatrick, D., Bucuvalas, M., Gold, J., & Vlahov, D. (2002). Psychological sequelae of the September 11 terrorist attacks in New York City. *New England Journal of Medicine, 346,* 982–987.

Gerrity, E. T., & Flynn, B. W. (1997). Mental health consequences of disasters. In E. K. Noji (Ed.), *The Public Health Consequences of Disasters* (pp. 101–121). New York: Oxford Press.

Herman, J. L. (1992). *Trauma and Recovery: The Aftermath of Violence from Domestic Abuse to Political Terror.* New York: Basic Books.

Imamura, K. (1995). Mental health in Japan. *Lancet, 346,* 509–510.

Inglesby, T. V., Henderson, S. D. A., Ascher, M. S., Eitzen, E., Friedlander, A. M., et al. (1999). Anthrax as a biological weapon. *Journal of the American Medical Association, 281,* 1735–1745.

Jacobs, G. A., & Kulkarni, N. (1999). Mental health responses to terrorism. *Psychiatric Annals, 29,* 376–380.

Janoff-Bulman, R., & Freize, I. H. (1983). A theoretical perspective for understanding reactions to victimization. *Journal of Social Issues, 39,* 1–17.

Jenkins, B. M. (1984, November). *The who, what, where, how, and why of terrorism.* Paper presented at the Detroit Police Department conference on urban terrorism, Detroit, Michigan, MI.

Jenkins, B. M. (1985). *International Terrorism: The Other World War.* Santa Monica, CA: Rand.

Kahneman, D., & Tversky, A. (1973). On the psychology of prediction. *Psychological Review, 80,* 237–251.

Kaniasty, K., Norris, F., & Murrell, S. A. (1995). Received and perceived social support following natural disaster. *Journal of Applied Social Psychology, 20,* 85–114.

Kidder, R. M. (1993). Unmasking terrorism: Manipulation of the media. In B. Schecterman, & M. Slann (Eds.), *Violence and Terrorism* (3rd ed., pp. 130–134). Guilford, CT: Guilford Publishing.

Koppel, T. (1993). Comment on media and terrorism. In B. Schecterman, & M. Slann (Eds.), *Violence and Terrorism* (3rd ed., p. 133). Guilford, CT: Guilford Publishing.

Krug, E. G., Kresnow, M. J., Peddicord, J. P., Dahlberg, L. L., Powell, K. E., Crosby, A. E., et al. (1998). Suicide after natural disasters. *New England Journal of Medicine, 338,* 373–378.

Lee, M. A. (1990). *Unreliable Sources: A Guide to Detecting Bias in Mass Media.* New York: Carol Publishing Group.

Lew, E. O., & Wetli, C. V. (1996). Mortality from hurricane Andrew. *Journal of Forensic Science, 41,* 449–452.

Lipton, E. (2001, April 19). In cold numbers, a census of Sept. 11 victims. *The New York Times,* p. 3.

Meselson, M, Guillemin, J., & Hugh-Jones, M. (1994). The Sverdlovsk anthrax outbreak of 1979. *Science, 266,* 1202–1208.

Murray, B. (2001). It exposed America's vulnerability. *Monitor on Psychology, 32.* Retrieved July 3, 2002 from www.apa.monitor/nov01/

Myers, D. G. (2001). Do we fear the right things? *APS Observer.* Retrieved July 3, 2002 from www. psychologicalscience.org/1201/

Ohbu, S., Yamashina, A., Takasu, N., Yamaguchi, T., Murai, T., Nakano, K., et al. (1997). Sarin poisoning on Tokyo subway. *Southern Medical Journal, 90,* 587–593.

Paton, D. (1999). Disaster business continuity: Promoting staff capability. *Disaster Prevention and Management, 8,* 127–133.

Paton, D., Smith, L. M., Violanti, J. M., & Eränen, L. (2000). Work related trauma stress: Risk, vulnerability and resilience. In J. M. Violanti, D. Paton, & C. Dunning (Eds.), *Posttraumatic Stress Intervention: Challenges, Issues and Perspectives* (pp. 187–202). Springfield, IL: Charles C Thomas.

Pfefferbaum, B., Seale, T. W., McDonald, N. B., Brandt, E. N., Rainwater, S. M., Maynard, B. T., et al. (2000). Posttraumatic stress two years after the Oklahoma City bombing in youths geographically distant from the explosion. *Psychiatry, 63,* 358–370.

Rosie, G. (1987). *The Dictionary of International Terrorism.* New York: Paragon House.

Schechterman, B., & Slann, M. (1993). *Violence and Terrorism.* Guilford, CT: Guilford Publishing.

Schmid, A. P. (1983). *Political Terrorism: A Research Guide to Concepts, Theories, Databases, and Literature.* New Brunswick, CT: Transaction.

Schmid, A. P., & DeGraff, J. F. A. (1982). *Violence as Communication.* Newbury Park, CA: Sage Publishing.

Scotti, J. R., Beach, B. K., Northrop, L. M. E., Rode, C. A., & Forsyth, J. P. (1995). The psychological impact of accidental injury. In J. R. Freedy, & S. E. Hobfall (Eds.), *Traumatic Stress: From Theory to Practice* (pp. 150–176). New York: Plenum.

Shuster, M. A., Stein, B. D., Jaycox, L. H., Collins, R. L., Marshall, G. N., Elliott, M. N., Zhou, A. J., & Kanouse, D. E. (2001). A national survey of stress reaction after the September 11, 2001, terrorist attacks. *New England Journal of Medicine, 345,* 1507–1512.

Slone, M. (2000). Responses to media coverage of terrorism. *Journal of Conflict Resolution, 44,* 508–522.

Smith, E. M., North, C. S., & Price, P. C. (1988). Response to technological accidents. In M. Lystad (Ed.), *Response to Mass Emergencies: Theory and Practice* (pp. 53–65). New York: Brunner/Mazel.

Solomon, S. D. (1992). Mental health effects of natural and human-made disasters. *PTSD Research Quarterly, 3,* 107.

Terr, L. C., Bloch, D. A., Michel, B. A., Shi, H., Reinhardt, J. A., & Metayer, S. A. (1999). Children's symptoms in the wake of Challenger: A field study of distant traumatic effects and an outline of related conditions. *American Journal of Psychiatry, 156,* 1536–1544.

US Congressional Office of Technology Assessment. (1993). *Proliferation of weapons of mass destruction* (Publication No. OTA-ISC-559). Washington, DC: US Government Printing Office.

Violanti, J. M. (1990). Posttrauma vulnerability: A proposed model. In J. W. Reese, J. M. Horn, & C. Dunning (Eds.), *Critical Incidents in Policing* (pp. 503–510). Washington, DC: US Government Printing Office.

Warheit, G. J., Zimmerman, R. S., Khoury, E. L., Vega, W. A., & Gil, A. G. (1996). Disaster related stresses, depressive signs and symptoms, and suicidal ideation among a multi-racial/ethnic sample of adolescents: A longitudinal analysis. *Journal of Child Psychology and Psychiatry, 37,* 435–444.

White, J. R. (1998). *Terrorism: An Introduction* (2nd ed.). New York: West/Wadsworth.

World Health Organization. (1970). *Health Aspects of Chemical and Biological Weapons.* Geneva, Switzerland: WHO.

WuDunn, S., Miller J., & Broad, W. (1998, May 26). How Japan germ terror alerted the world. *New York Times,* p. 4.

Yehuda, R. (2002). Post-Traumatic Stress Disorder. *New England Journal of Medicine, 346,* 108–114.

Zilinskas, R. A. (1997). Iraq's biological weapons: The past as the future? *Journal of the American Medical Association, 278,* 418–424.

Zimbardo, P. (2001). *The psychology of terrorism: Mind games and healing.* Retrieved July 3, 2002 from American Psychological Association Web site: www.apa.org/science/

Chapter 14

MANAGING TRAUMATIC STRESS IN PROTECTIVE SERVICES: RISK, RESILIENCE, AND VULNERABILITY

Douglas Paton, John M. Violanti, Christine Dunning, and Leigh M. Smith

All too often, adverse psychological outcomes following exposure to traumatic or critical incidents are treated as a *fait accompli*. While the current volume does not deny the possibility of protective services professionals experiencing adverse stress reactions, it does argue that we can make choices regarding the psychological consequences of exposure to such events.

Growing evidence for the existence of loss and growth outcomes following exposure to critical incidents makes it imperative that the ability to influence the outcomes experienced is acknowledged and that frameworks within which choices can be made are identified. The risk-management paradigm was used here to frame the process of making choices. Furthermore, the notion of "making choices" implies a proactive approach, one that is fundamental to the effective exercise of organizational duty of care.

Risk management affords protective services organizations an opportunity to focus on the primary prevention of traumatic stress. Primary prevention strategies are designed to develop capabilities to prevent or contain adverse reactions and facilitate a positive resolution *prior to* exposure. The risk-management approach described here stands in contrast to contemporary mental health practices that have blurred the distinction between primary and secondary prevention (De Soir, 2003). Secondary prevention refers to actions undertaken when a person has developed a condition or when he or she is at risk for further health damage. While we are not arguing that secondary intervention is redundant, it should be complemented by strategies that focus on reducing risk in the first place.

To make judgments about traumatic stress risk, protective services personnel must gather two basic pieces of information. One concerns the likelihood of an event occurring. The other concerns the consequences. The interaction between these factors provides an estimate of risk. To manage risk, we thus need to change the values of one or the other of these factors. It is generally outside the ability of protective services agencies to influence the likelihood of occurrence of potentially traumatic events. They can, however, make choices about the consequences of exposure to such events. To make these choices, we need to understand at what points risk reduction can occur. Fundamentally, intervention can take place at one or more of three points. This book is primarily concerned with one of these points, psychological hazards. Psychological hazards are defined as the agents, processes, and expectations capable of threatening psychological integrity. A knowledge of psychological hazards is thus fundamental to understanding risk.

These hazards, or risk factors, have typically been identified as originating within the experience of the traumatic event. Indeed, as Schmuckler (Chapter 2), Gehrke and Violanti (Chapter 6), Paton and Hannan (Chapter 7), Bartone (Chapter 8) have discussed, many psychological hazards can indeed arise within this context. These include, for example, exposure to physical danger, recovering human remains, making urgent and complex decisions, and working under high time pressures. However, risk can also be traced to developmental history (Samuels, Chapter 5); professional socialization and expectation (Gehrke & Violanti, Chapter 6; Paton, Taylor & McFarlane, Chapter 9; Bicknell Chapter 10); organizational practices such as selection (Dunning, Chapter 3); and organizational and family environments (Sevastos, Chapter 11; Shakespeare-Finch & Gow, Chapter 12). Consequently, risk assessment must extend beyond analysis of the event experience per se to include the contextual factors that surround any specific experience. Indeed, there is growing evidence that these contextual factors may represent equally important, if not more important, predictors of adverse and growth outcomes alike (Hart & Cooper, 2000; Huddleston, Stephens, & Paton, in press). This evidence supports the conclusion not only that the latter factors must be accommodated in traumatic stress risk management, but also that their pervasive nature prior to, during, and after exposure provides a very strong indicator of a need and a basis for primary prevention strategies to be developed and implemented. For example, organizational and family dynamics are not amenable to change through any sort of brief intervention. They require primary prevention in the form of change or the development of family-friendly policies.

In addition to providing a catalyst for organizational and environmental change and development, a knowledge of psychological hazards is important in several other respects. They represent the event characteristics, demands, and operational practices that should be modeled in simulations to create realistic training scenarios (Paton & Flin, 1999). Knowledge of hazards provides the context within which the validity of selection measures (Dunning, Chapter 3) can be assessed. Knowledge of hazards emanating from work and nonwork environments provides a framework for organizational analysis and the subsequent development of appropriate management and response procedures and practices and for the development of support resources and practices. Hazard information should also be accommodated in postevent intervention (Dunning, 1999).

However, psychological hazards represent only one of three components of the "consequences" facet of the risk-management process. Estimates of consequences, and thus risk, will be a function of how hazards interact with resilience and vulnerability factors (at personal, group, and environmental levels). Information on psychological hazards thus not only has a direct input into understanding risk; it also identifies what resilience factors protective services personnel and their organizations must possess if they are to respond positively to these hazards. Such information also helps identify what personal, group, and environmental characteristics are capable of increasing vulnerability to adverse consequences. Thus, comprehensive risk management requires an ability to estimate all three components.

The assessment of resilience and vulnerability may require going beyond the more straightforward process of identifying specific factors (although this remains a core aspect of risk assessment). For example, Gehrke and Violanti (Chapter 5) and Sevastos (Chapter 11) discuss the need to view protective factors in a contingent light. Gehrke and Violanti illustrate how social networks can, depending on size, act to ameliorate stress or contribute to increased susceptibility to adverse stress reactions. Sevastos (Chapter 11) illustrates a similar contingent process with reference to Warr's (1999) "Vitamin Model." Thus, it may not just be the presence or absence of specific factors that affects outcome. These observations reiterate not only the importance of the systematic assessment of resilience and vulnerability factors, but also the need for their more critical analysis before any decision regarding their specific capacity, relative to the psychological hazards likely to be encountered, or their contingent influences can be made. A start has been made regarding the identification of the resilience factors that should be subject to a more stringent analysis (Paton, Violanti, & Smith, 2003). A similar exercise must be conducted for the personal, group, and environmental factors that might affect vulnerability to adverse reactions.

This text provides a contemporary, theoretically rigorous and, where possible, an empirically supported review of traumatic stress hazards. This knowledge can provide an important input into the development of strategies capable of proactively mitigating traumatic stress reactions and promoting the development of personal and professional growth in people who have been exposed to disaster and traumatic incidents.

Hazards arise in several contexts and from several events, as well as from professional and organizational sources. Knowledge of these hazards provides a basis for risk-reduction activities involving, for example, personnel selection, training, professional socialization, and the development of organizational practices, procedures, and systems necessary to mitigate risk and promote well-being. Armed with this knowledge and with an acceptance of the fact that it is within the remit of any protective services organization to make choices regarding the traumatic stress risk, organizations can make more informed decisions regarding what constitutes acceptable levels of risk and where responsibility for its management should lie (Paton, 2003). The process outlined here facilitates the application of risk-management principles to mental health and physical hazards alike.

Because risk management is an iterative process, assessment of unacceptable levels of risk provides the foundation for risk-reduction strategies to determine risk-management priorities by evaluating and comparing the level of risk against predetermined standards, target risk levels, or other criteria. The latter can be based on managing one or more of the components (hazards, resilience, vulnerability) of the "consequences" facet of the risk equation. Currently, risk is typically perceived as emanating from the person-event transaction. However, because the components that contribute to "consequences" comprise personal, group, and environmental elements, the risk-reduction process will also include strategies that transfer responsibility for managing risk. This means that organizations and professions must acknowledge their contribution to risk and accept responsibility for its management accordingly.

REFERENCES

De Soir, E. (2003). The CRASH-model for psychosocial crisis intervention: From peer driven early intervention to professional care and therapeutic action with military and emergency services. *Forum, 8,* 27–51.

Dunning, C. (1999). Post-intervention strategies to reduce police trauma: A paradigm shift. In J. M. Violanti, & D. Paton (Eds.), *Police Trauma: Psychological Aftermath of Civilian Combat* (pp. 269–292). Springfield, IL: Charles C Thomas.

Hart, P. M., & Cooper, C. L. (2001) Occupational stress: Toward a more integrated framework. In N. Anderson, D. S. Ones, H. K. Sinangil, & C. Viswesvaren (Eds.), *International Handbook of Work and Organizational Psychology, Vol.2: Organizational Psychology.* London: Sage Publications.

Huddleston, L. M., Stephens, C., & Paton, D. (in press). An evaluation of traumatic and organisational experiences on the psychological health of New Zealand police recruits. *Work.*

Paton, D. (2003). *Emergency Management: Conceptual Issues.* Palmerston North, New Zealand: NSATS.

Paton, D., & Flin, R. (1999). Disaster Stress: An emergency management perspective. *Disaster Prevention and Management, 8,* 261–267.

Paton, D, Violanti, J. M., & Smith, L. M. (2003). *Promoting Capabilities to Manage Post-traumatic Stress: Perspectives on Resilience.* Springfield, IL: Charles C Thomas.

Warr, P. B. (1999). Well-being and the workplace. In D. Kaheman, E. Diener, & N. Schwarz (Eds.), *Well-being: The Foundation of Hedonic Psychology* (pp. 392–412). New York: Russell Sage Foundation.

SUBJECT INDEX

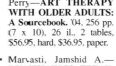
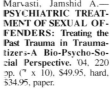

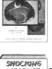

 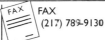 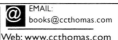 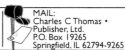